Dr. Sebi's

Alkaline and Anti-Inflammatory Diet for Beginners

Reduce Inflammation and Boost Immunity With the Original Healing Treatments.
| Alkaline Recipes, 30-Days Detox Plan, and More!

Suzanne Scarrett

"Make food your medicine and medicine your food"

(Hippocrates)

Table of Content

SALAD RECIPES 89

DESSERT AND SNACK RECIPES 100

30- DAY MEAL PLAN 112

CONCLUSION 115

Suzanne Scarrett

Hi, I'm Suzanne.

Thank you for purchasing my book.

I invite you to visit my website, which I update regulary

www.suzannescarrett.com

I am genuinely happy and proud of everything my team and I can do and deliver to our customers.

You will find several recipes with images and articles about nutrition and health. Furthermore, I am at your complete disposal to receive any advice or request you want to write privately.

If you have the pleasure, you can download a PDF guide completely free of charge to fight problems related to acidity, gastritis, conjunctivitis, constipation, diarrhea, eczema, fever, indigestion, and many other topics in a completely natural way.

My team and I are experts in this subject, and we would be delighted if we could help you or someone close to you to solve their health issues.

Just scan the QR code below with your smartphone.

All that remains is to wish you much joy and serenity by reading this book.

Thank you   *Suzanne*

SUZANNE SCARRETT

Introduction

Dr. Sebi is a physician, botanist, organic chemist, and naturalist. He has studied herbs in North, Central, and South America, Africa, and the Caribbean and has developed a new methodology and system related to the repair of the human body with herbs that have established themselves as real estate in more than 30 years of experience.

On November 26, 1933, Dr. Sebi was born Alfredo Bowman in Ilanga, Honduras, Spain. Dr. Sebi is a self-taught man. His adorable grandmother, "Mama Hay," encouraged him to respect life's experiences. The beginning of the game and her perception of the stream and the forested area, combined with her grandmother's guidance, helped Sebi establish himself to be submissive to the Truth in his future life. Sebi did dedicate over 30 years of his life to creating an interesting technique.

Dr. Sebi accepted the Western way to deal with malady to be incapable. He held that bodily fluid and acridity — rather microscopic organisms and infections, for instance — caused malady.

A fundamental hypothesis behind the diet is that malady can just make do in acidic situations. The point of the diet is to accomplish an alkaline state in the body to prevent or destroy illness.

Dr. Sebi planned this diet for any individual who wishes to normally fix or prevent infection and improve their general wellbeing without depending on the regular Western medication.

Advantages of the alkaline diet

The Alkaline diet is considered by many experts to be a real panacea for our body. This is because its principles are very ancient, and its applications are many. Just think that in prehistoric times, when modern medicine did not exist, herbs and spices were used to cure all the ills of that time. Of course, today, our society has profoundly changed, but the general principles on which this diet is based are still valid and scientifically proven.

For these reasons, knowing thoroughly and correctly how the alkaline diet works will help you to properly purify your body and, of course, to lose weight. In addition, we will eliminate certain toxic foods and introduce others that have natural powers for your body.

Therefore, the Alkaline Diet is a valid alternative to traditional treatments and takes us directly to the future.

Finally, the alkaline diet will allow you to become more aware of the nature of each food that enters your diet and what you can find every day in a supermarket.

The healing power of plants

That's right. Most alkaline foods are of plant origin, and using them in our diet allows us to achieve extraordinary results.

The mix and union of several vegetables in each meal allow you to assimilate a vast amount of beneficial substances. It will enable you to stay in shape in the short and long term.

Natural-chemical substances have always been considered a true panacea. The great thing is that they are adequately metabolized by your body and do not leave any form of residue, unlike the chemicals contained in some common drugs that instead leave traces and residues over time and accumulate in the body.

Therefore, vegetables have miraculous substances that help us feel good and find the energy our body needs to face the day in the best way.

In fact, are to be preferred foods mainly of vegetal origin and, above all, not too much processed as opposed to the most refined foods or those processed by human activity. This second class of foods, in fact, has undergone one or more dietary processes that indeed make food more delicious, but at the same time make it more toxic and harmful, especially if taken regularly in the long run.

The extraordinary universe of vegetable foods is ready to wait for us. New technologies are also available at a low price and just a few meters away from us.

Intermittent Fasting

Intermittent fasting is another form of healing for your body.

In general, I recommend everyone to try intermittent fasting at least twice a year for a given period to thoroughly cleanse the body.

The first recommendation I want to give you now is that performing any form of fasting is better if you follow the advice of an expert or a doctor. This way, you will know what can be healthy for your body and whatnot.

Intermittent fasting is based on a simple principle. When our body is in a post-prandial phase (i.e., away from meals), it can produce metabolic energy from fat reserves. It can cope with all the functions of basal metabolism.

Entering a fasting state is not easy. You must first prepare your body physically (by first introducing the right foods) and spiritually.

For this reason, each of us follows an individual path with varying times and rhythms.

The end result will be a true transformation of your body and soul. In fact, hearing feedback from people who have performed this practice, they describe it as "a spiritual renewal practice" or a "deep purification."

This feedback is accurate in that the body has literally rid itself of toxic substances accumulated over time.

Who can perform fasting?

As powerful and rewarding as it can be, fasting cannot be performed freely by everyone. For example, if you are on a particular drug therapy that requires certain foods in your diet, then you cannot perform fasting.

Again, if you are a pregnant woman or a woman who has just given birth, you cannot perform fasting.

In conclusion, as mentioned before, always follow the guidelines that your doctor gives you and do not try to thwart the nature of your body.

To whom is it recommended?

Fasting can be safely recommended to a healthy person who performs regular physical activity and a person who wants to lose weight quickly. In addition, it is looking for new emotions and forms of purification.

How to start?

The beginning of fasting is never too easy, especially in the first hours. To get the best start in the meantime is necessary to establish a start and end date of fasting on our calendar. You can very well start with one or two days, or even skip a meal (such as breakfast or dinner) to put the night's rest in the middle of the fast.

This practice is also highly recommended for older people who have a slightly different social life than someone in their 40s or 50s.

Remember, however, that fasting is a dietary practice and should be tailored to your life. For example, a skilled worker performing physical labor is unlikely to follow a relatively long period of fasting. On the other hand, an employee behind a computer screen has other physiological needs and different energy expenditures for his activity.

To start, however, it is necessary to follow for at least 14 days a diet rich in fiber vegetables (raw or cooked depending on the season in which you are) and significantly reduce carbohydrates.

Regarding the intake of fats instead, there is straightforward advice. They can be taken in varying amounts (as long as they are not coupled to simple sugars as in sweets). Still, you should prefer the healthier and unsaturated ones.

After 14 days have passed, you can begin to slowly reduce the portions of your meals until you eliminate the whole meal.

Remember that during the whole fasting phase and in its preparation, it is necessary to hydrate your body to the maximum. All hormones involved in metabolism use water for their proper functioning. So do not neglect the intake of liquids or herbal teas.

What are the best times to start?

I highly recommend starting with a day or two and jotting down any emotions or sensations your body sends you. To create a new fasting practice is necessary to repeat the diet followed for the 14 days described above and gradually extend the days of fasting duration. It is not required to follow very long periods of fasting; they could even bring your body to a state of suffering. Instead, it is healthier to practice short periods of fasting close to each other so that your body slowly eliminates the toxic waste accumulated over time.

Remember to constantly monitor your weight; excessive and rapid weight loss is not suitable for your body.

Benefits?

The advantages of practicing fasting are many and go beyond the physical aspects.

Having completed a phase of fasting (short or long) brings considerable benefits to your person's general state of health. For example, you will feel better and have better relationships with others.

Fasting also has an economic benefit. By taking in very few foods, you will not be forced to spend more money to follow this path.

The resulting weight loss will bring so many benefits to your body, and you will regain new forms of energy.

Dr. Sebi's Recommended Method for Combating Diseases

Dr. Sebi employed the process of cleansing and detoxification of the body, and he concluded that this method is a vital tool necessary in dealing with any form of illness in the body.

Detoxification of the body helps removes mucus stored in the body and helps remove surplus acidic materials, thus making the body free from disease-causing organisms. He employed the use of herbs that are essential in re-energizing and revitalizing the body.

Other Home Remedies

These home remedies are made by Dr. Sebi's approved products. Some of the products are already in your kitchen cabinet, waiting for you to use them. These products can help you reduce itching, swelling, stinging, etc. However, what we have in our diet plays an important role in the healing process of herpes simplex. This is the reason why Dr. Sebi's diet is recommended for the treatment of herpes.

Some foods help to strengthen the immune system. If the immune system is strong enough, the body can easily fight the herpes simplex virus without any medication. Studies have shown that our diet is important in the prevention of disease breakout.

The foods we eat are very important. Some of these foods and nutrients that can help the body to naturally heal from herpes are.

Vegetables

Dr. Sebi's diet has a lot of veggies one can turn to for antioxidant supply. Antioxidants help to boost the immune in the body. So, eating a lot of vegetables can help to fight against the herpes simplex virus. Moreover, these vegetables contain high amounts of lysine, an amino acid that helps to fight the herpes virus.

Vitamin C

Studies suggest that vitamin C plays a vital role in the healing of herpes and other viral diseases. Dr. Sebi's diet has a lot of fruits and vegetables packed with vitamin C. Some of these fruits and vegetables are orange, strawberries, papaya, peppers, mango, etc.

The Cleansing Journey

Making the stomach safe is linked with cleansing. The digestive system is the system from the body that receives its nutrients from. It becomes inefficient in performing out its tasks as it gets unstable. In the stomach, the pile-up of the dump will turn poisonous, contributing to pain and disease. Bloating is among the symptoms of a dysfunctional stomach. When the body cannot get rid of waste, that's due to the accumulation of gas. The food continues to decompose then. Food, as meant by default, must be natural and organic.

There are both positive and destructive microbes in the digestive system. It contributes to problems if the equilibrium of such bacteria is disrupted. Purging, in which a laxative is used to eliminate human waste, parasites, and other such unnecessary material, is the essential method of cleansing. The concern with this technique, though, is that it would be non-selective and clears up the benefits with the harmful. It may also be harmful since, during the phase, you may lose extra water, which would make you drained. One of its reasons the body system gets a strip of toxic chemicals is to consume lots of water.

A vice president and dietician of the Sports Education Society, Marie Spano, claims that workouts and adequate sleep play a vital role in making you function on the detox regimen.

Through curing the gut by taking note of what goes through it, a healthy way to detox is to practice regularly. It's considered fast food, and it doesn't have the nutrition your body requires. Instead, clogging things up appears to screw with the digestive tract. Soy, gluten, dairy, sugar, and caffeine-containing foods can be removed and substituted with unprocessed agricultural substitutes and additives.

The method of cleansing is not only complete with the clearance of waste from the digestive system. By supplying nutritious food that makes the gut function at its peak, it should be cured. This requires balanced food that has adequate nutrition, which tends to maintain the safe levels of microbes in the stomach, such as good bacteria—organic beverages, such as unflavored probiotic yogurt, often aid.

The Detox Route

Another approach to clear the body of destructive chemicals is to detox. Normally, through the liver, skin, and kidneys, the body requires the removal of pollutants. The contributions of these organs can be strengthened by Detox. So, what toxins are attacked by the process? For example, there are contaminants in the atmosphere you breathe in that make their way through your bloodstream, where they settle and create pain. Chemicals such as toxins, preservatives, and additives are still used in a few products. During this time, meat must be avoided.

One of the actors whose detox was performed with is Gwyneth Paltrow. Over a 21-day duration, it is circulated. It's named The Safe Method by the psychiatrist who developed it. To clear the body of contaminants, he recommends a diet of shakes, nutritious foods, and vitamins—any of his patient's record post-program weight loss.

Your skin is often loaded with a mixture of chemicals hidden on the lotions of creams and other products you use. Often, the organs associated with detoxifying get overloaded. The detox can be supported by ingredients such as lemon, garlic, spinach, pineapple, and ginger. As several may have detrimental consequences, you can address them with a nutritionist. For starters, garlic thins the blood, which may threaten someone whose blood doesn't easily coagulate. Health supplements, too, aid enhance the health of the liver and kidneys.

What are Some Detoxification/Cleansing Approaches?

Many detoxification programs are offered in an integrative health care model. The following areas are some strategies you can follow to eliminate toxins in your body:

- *Exercise/movement*
- Body-mind balance (yoga, meditation, breathing, prayer)
- Pure/alkaline water
- *Diet*
- *Fasting*
- *Juicing*

- *Supplements*
- Detox Massages and Body Scrubs
- Infrared Sauna
- Lymphatic drainage
- Ozone therapy (autohemotherapy)
- Detox infusions
- Colon Hydrotherapy
- *Osteopathy*

ALKALINE AND ANTI-INFLAMMATORY TIPS

Why Detox Your Body

Practically, there have been 8 ways in which contaminants impact our bodies that need detoxification.

Pollutants Poison Enzymes Such That They Don't Act Correctly

Our body systems are the engines of enzymes. To generate molecules, create energy, and build cell structures, and physiological response relies on enzymes. Toxins harm enzymes and thereby impair myriad body functions, such as inhibiting hemoglobin development in the blood or reducing the ability of the body to resist free-radical damage, which accelerates aging.

Structural Minerals Are Displaced by Pollutants, Resulting in Weakened Bones

For lifetime mobility, people must retain good bone density. There is indeed a twofold consequence as toxins replace the calcium contained in the bone: weakened skeletal systems and enhanced toxins, generated through bone degradation, circulated around the body.

Organs Are Impaired by Toxins

Nearly all tissues and structures are damaged by toxins. The Toxin Cure, my novel, concentrates primarily on detox organs. Your detoxification can backfire because the body would remain acidic if the digestive system, liver, and kidneys are too contaminated that they are not able to cleanse efficiently.

DNA, which raises the risk of aging and degeneration, is impaired by toxins.

Many widely used contaminants, phthalates and estrogen that are poorly detoxified, and benzene-containing materials, damage DNA.

Toxins Change the Expression of Genes

To respond to shifts in our parts of the body and the outside world, our genes turn off and on. But certain contaminants trigger our DNA in unhealthy ways or block them.

Toxins Destroy the Membranes of Cells Such That They Do Not Respond Properly

In cell membranes, "signaling" exists in the body. Harm to such membrane inhibits them from obtaining essential stimuli, such as insulin that does not warn the cells to consume more sugar, or body tissues that do not respond to the magnesium message to relax.

Toxins Interact and Create Imbalances in the Hormones

Toxins trigger chemicals, disrupt, imitate, and destroy them. For example, arsenic disrupts the cells' thyroid hormone receptors because the cells do not obtain the signal through thyroid hormones, which trigger the metabolism to rev up. Inexplicable exhaustion is the consequence.

Toxins, finally, but not only, potentially inhibit the detoxification potential, and it's the worst concern of all. It's tougher when you're already unhealthy and must detoxify urgently, even when you're not unhealthy. In other words, your hard-working cleansing mechanism is more likely to run below average exactly as you will need your recovery systems more (to fix health problems). And why? Since your recovery potential has been exhausted by the strong toxic burden you still bear. That is right. The more contaminants your body is burdened with, the stronger the harm to the detoxification processes in the body.

That's why it's such an essential challenge to rebuild your detox body parts and your detox mechanisms with them. The net effect is that contaminants will then be freely expelled by the body.

Helpful Ideas for Detox

While the use of such detox diets to eliminate toxins from the body is not confirmed by current evidence, some changes in diet and lifestyle habits can help reduce the toxin load and support the detoxification mechanism of your body.

- *Eat foods containing Sulphur.* Sulfur-high foods such as broccoli, onions, as well as garlic improve the removal of heavy metals such as mercury.

- *Try chlorella.* As per animal research, a chlorella is indeed a form of algae that has several vital nutrients and may boost the absorption of contaminants such as heavy metals.

- *Using cilantro to spice dishes.* Cilantro improves the excretion of many pollutants, including heavy metals such as lead and contaminants such as phthalates and insecticides.

- *Glutathione Help.* Consuming foods high in Sulphur, such as meat, broccoli, and garlic, may increase the role of glutathione, the significant antioxidant the body creates that is strongly engaged in purification.

- *Turn to clean items that are safe.* You will reduce your sensitivity to possibly harmful substances by preferring natural cleaning materials like vinegar and baking soda above synthetic cleaning agents.

- *Choose natural treatment for the body.* Your susceptibility to toxins will also be minimized by utilizing natural deodorants, shampoos, cosmetics, moisturizers, as well as other personal care items.

Dr. Sebi Products to Boost Immune System to Help in the Cure of Herpes

In this chapter, the products that mainly focus on the immune system and how to reduce inflammation are mentioned. These are basically herbal teas or nutritional supplements. They are being used widely for the betterment of health and well-being. As all diseases are the outcome of mucus, acidity, and a weak immune system, these products will help you to improve these specific areas of well-being.

The African Bio-Mineral Treatment Method studies and recognizes the mechanisms of sickness, not only the effects. In addition, it found that mucus is the source of the disorder. Inside the body, where mucus has been collected, an illness may appear. While the natural food compounds of the vegetation cells were engineered to remove mucus from a specific region of the body, it is often important to clean the body as a whole. The nature in which they function to purify and nourish the whole body is what renders the compounds special.

We have been active in restoring pathologies through this method. As the herbs included have such a natural background, 14 days after they have been initially taken, the compounds also unleash their cleaning properties. Adhering to the therapeutic recommendations given by Dr. Sebi is an equally significant feature of the African Bio-Mineral treatment. To maintain optimum wellness, our herbal compounds acting in combination with dietary improvements would give the body the correct climate. Also, please notice that if a meal is not mentioned in these sections, you are highly encouraged not to consume it. In addition, we notice that consuming a gallon of water recommended by Dr. Sebi every day tends to achieve the African Bio-Mineral Treatment's most valuable outcomes.

Dr. Sebi's Foods

Who is Dr. Sebi?

Alfredo Darlington Bowman is an African herbalist who developed an alkaline plant diet that is based on bio-mineral balance theory. Though he is not a certified medical doctor or a Ph.D. holder, he is widely known as Dr. Sebi.

His diet is named after his popular name, The Dr. Sebi Diet. His diet was developed for those that wish to naturally detox their body for total wellness and prevent diseases by eating approved healthy plant foods.

Dr. Sebi claimed that our body is protected from diseases when it is in an alkaline state. According to him, the acidic state of the body and mucus buildup in the body are the major causes of various diseases.

Though there is no scientific backup, Dr. Sebi claimed that his diet has the potential to cure lupus, sickle cell anemia, AIDS, and leukemia. He believes his diet could completely restore alkalinity in the body and detoxify the whole body.

Dr. Sebi's diet is regarded as a vegan diet since it is a completely plant-based diet. No animal product is allowed in the diet.

Dr. Sebi claimed that this diet can make the body heal itself completely from diseases. Though there is no scientific proof for this, a lot of people who are on the diet have attested to the claim.

As a result, Dr. Sebi's diet is ranked one of the most popular diets in 2019.

Why Is Dr. Sebi's Diet Successful?

Dr. Sebi's alkaline diet is a plant-based diet that helps to eliminate toxic wastes from the body and rejuvenate body cells.

The alkaline diet relies strictly on a list of plant foods and products approved by Dr. Sebi. Through his diet, Dr. Sebi did great wonders in people's lives, cured many diseases, and revived complicated health conditions. In fact, it is one of the best plant-based diets. It was listed as one of the most popular diets in 2019.

If we can eat delicious meals and free our body from diseases, what again are we looking for? Dr. Sebi's diet can help you detox your body completely, including mucus removal, liver cleansing, diabetes reversal, cancer treatment, lupus, and herpes cure, etc. Learn how to eat good foods, and you may not need medications to stay healthy.

You don't need medications to cleanse mucus from your body when you can easily get rid of it naturally by drinking and eating the right foods. By so doing, you can simply prevent and/or manage high blood pressure. The foods to take good care of your condition can be found in the nearest local grocery store.

Prepare your mind and stock your kitchen with the right foods from Dr. Sebi Approved List. Then follow the instructions in the book to help you quit smoking.

Key Points About Dr. Sebi's Diet

There are essential points you must consider before trying Dr. Sebi's diet. These points are described below:

Doctor Sebi's diet consists of all the types of foods you desire except for animal products.

His foods are alkaline grains, alkaline vegetables, alkaline fruits, alkaline nuts, alkaline tea, alkaline seeds, natural sweeteners, and alkaline curative herbs.

Doctor Sebi's diets are most effective in fighting different types of diseases. Hence, his diets prevent prophylactics and cure diseases.

Doctor Sebi's diet can help sustain a healthy lifestyle.

Dr. Sebi's diet helps in revitalizing, energizing, and rejuvenating the body.

Dieters who truly inculcate the use of the Sebi diets testify that the diets have done great work in their bodies.

He claimed that all infections grow properly in a mucus accumulated environment. He concluded that alkaline diets responsible for detoxification could help remove this mucus.

Again, he believed that removing excess mucus in the body via detoxification would help you eliminate any disease in your body.

Individuals who believe that good health is their utmost priority inculcate the habit of following the Sebi diets. They make you look clean and healthy.

Dr. Sebi's diet is solely based on plants and supplements approved by Dr. Sebi.

The diet guide can be found on his website. The simple rules to follow on Dr. Sebi diet are.

- Only foods and products listed in the nutritional guide are to be consumed.

- You must drink at least 1 gallon of water every day (that is about 3.8 liters).

- If you are on any medication, you must take your Dr. Sebi supplements at least one hour before your medication.

- You don't take alcohol.

- You must not eat any animal products.

- Don't use the microwave to prepare your food.

- Only consume naturally grown grains as listed in the guide. No wheat product is allowed.

- No seedless fruit and no canned food are permitted.

Moreover, you are expected to be using Dr. Sebi's supplements to support your diet.

How Does Dr. Sebi Classify Food?

He classified the foods list into six classes. These classes are:

Living Foods

These foods are not dead without consuming them. All live foods do not contain toxic components when they are left to undergo fermentation.

Moreso, living foods do not undergo destruction when they are not in their environment. The materials required for digestion are embedded in living food, which contains almost the same pH as water (pH 7). Examples are green vegetables, fruits that ripen from the tree, grain, and many others.

Raw Foods

These are living foods that have already undergone processing and they are undercooked. They are foods that are dried with the use of direct sunlight.

These foods also contain many components needed for the digestion process and are spoiled within a short time if not adequately dried. Examples are dried fruits and vegetables, vegetables that roasted, fermented fruit juice, and many others.

Dead Foods

These are foods that, when fermented, become toxic, and have a prolonged life span. They are overdone and over-processed foods. Examples are deep-fried foods, synthetic foods, alcohols, sugars, and many others.

Hybrid Foods

They are foods that are not naturally grown but are cross-pollinated. The vitamins and mineral levels cannot be quantified, and they cannot be produced in the wild. Hybrid foods are mostly sugars that are not recognized by the digestive system. Examples are cows, pigs, chicken, sausage roll, and many others.

Genetically Modified Foods (GMO)

These are food improved by the man with the use of genetics. They mostly damage immunity in humans. These foods form an abnormal attitude in humans and cause genetic consequences in the body. Examples are grown hastily, weather-resistant foods such as corn, yeast, brown rice, and many others.

Drugs

Many Drugs are dangerous and harmful to the body. They are incredibly toxic and acidic. Most of them are extracted and are synthetic. Examples are cocaine, sugar, all prescription drugs, heroin, and many others.

Dr. Sebi's Recommended Nutritional Food Lists

Spices and Seasonings

- Achiote
- Habanero
- Savory
- Oregano
- Basil
- Thyme
- Pure sea salt
- Powdered granulated seaweed
- Sage
- Tarragon
- Cloves
- Dill

- Bay Leaf
- Cayenne
- Sweet Basil
- Onion Powder
- Herbs List
- Cayenne
- Dill
- Oregano
- Basil
- Onion powder
- Pure sea salt

Vegetable List

- Bell pepper
- Chayote
- Cucumber
- Wild arugula
- Avocado
- Green amaranth
- Dandelion greens
- Turnip greens
- Wakame
- Onions
- Arame
- Cherry and plum tomato
- Dulse
- Garbanzo beans

- Izote flower and leaf
- Olives
- Purslane verdolaga
- Squash
- Okra
- Tomatillo
- Kale
- Mushrooms except for shitake
- Hijiki
- Nopales
- Nori
- Zucchini
- Watercress
- Lettuce except for iceberg

Herbal Teas List

- Ginger
- Fennel
- Tila
- Chamomile
- Elderberry
- Burdock
- Red Raspberry

Alkaline Sugar Lists

- 100% Pure Agave Syrup from cactus
- Dried Date Sugar

Dr. Sebi's Fruit List

- Apples
- Bananas
- Berries
- Cantaloupe
- Cherries
- Currants
- Dates
- Figs
- Grapes
- Limes
- Mango
- Melons
- Orange
- Papayas
- Peaches
- Pears
- Plums
- Prickly Pear
- Prunes
- Raisins
- Soft Jelly Coconuts
- Soursoups

Dr. Sebi's Herbal Teas

- Burdock
- Chamomile
- Elderberry
- Fennel
- Ginger
- Red Raspberry
- Tila

Dr. Sebi's Alkaline Grains

- Amaranth
- Fonio
- Kamut
- Quinoa
- Rye
- Spelt
- Tef
- Wild Rice

Foods to Avoid

Acidic Foods

Acidic foods are not good for the healing of herpes. Foods with high acidic levels are not good for herpes infection. These foods can open the cold sore before it heals, and this prolongs the healing period. So, avoid foods like juice, soda, etc. You may consider taking water as a substitute until the sickness heals.

Arginine

Chocolate and some other foods high in L-arginine should be avoided. L-arginine is known to prolong the healing of the herpes virus.

Sugar

Instead of taking added sugar, one can easily go for oranges, mango, bananas, etc. Added sugar is usually converted to acid in the body.

Processed Foods

By maintaining a low level of oxidative stress, you can naturally quicken the healing process. Processed foods may promote oxidative stress due to synthetic preservatives.

Alcohol

Studies have shown that alcohol can suppress white blood cells. This means that alcohol can make the body susceptible to infections.

Note to the Reader

If you have found this book helpful, I invite you to leave a review directly on the Amazon page. Just scan the QR code on this page with your smartphone.

If you have any other requests or particular questions, you can freely contact me via mail.

scarrett.diet@outlook.com

Remember to also look at my site, I upgrade regulary.

www.suzannescarrett.com

You can also find me on Facebook and if you wish, put a like on my personal page.

Enjoy your life. I wish you much joy and serenity.

RECIPES

Breakfast

Crunchy Quinoa Meal

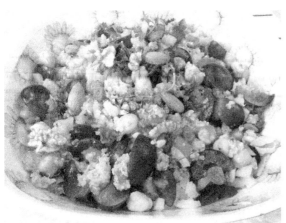

Preparation Time: 5 minutes | **Cooking Time:** 25 minutes | **Servings:** 2

Ingredients:

o   3 cups of coconut milk

o   1 cup quinoa, rinsed

o   1/8 teaspoon ground cinnamon

o   1 cup raspberry

o   ½ cup chopped coconuts

Directions:

1.   Add milk into a saucepan and boil over high heat. Then put the quinoa in the milk and boil it again.

2.   Let it simmer for 15 minutes, on low heat, until milk is reduced. Stir in cinnamon and mix well.

3.   Cover and cook for 8 minutes until the milk is completely absorbed. Add raspberry and cook for 30 seconds. Serve and enjoy.

Nutrition

Calories: 271 Fat: 3.7g Carbs: 54g Protein: 6.5g Fiber: 3.5g

Coconut Pancakes

Preparation Time: 5 minutes | **Cooking Time:** 15 minutes | **Servings:** 4

Ingredients:

o   1 cup coconut flour

o   2 tablespoons arrowroot powder

o   teaspoon baking powder

o   1 cup of coconut milk

o   3 tablespoons coconut oil

Directions:

1.   Mix all dry Ingredients in a medium container. Add coconut milk and 2 tablespoons coconut oil. Mix well. Melt a teaspoon coconut oil in a skillet.

2.   Pour a ladle of the batter into the skillet and swirl the pan to spread it into a smooth pancake. Cook for 3 minutes on low heat until firm.

3.   Flip the pancake and fry for another 2 to 3 minutes until golden brown—Cook more pancakes using the remaining batter. Serve.

Nutrition:

Calories: 377 Fat: 14.9g Carbs: 60.7g Protein: 6.4g Fiber: 1.4g

Quinoa Porridge

Preparation Time: 5 minutes | **Cooking Time:** 25 minutes | **Servings:** 2

Ingredients:

o   2 cups of coconut milk

o   1 cup quinoa, rinsed

o   1/8 teaspoon ground cinnamon

o   1 cup (1/2 pint) fresh blueberries

Directions:

1.   Boil coconut milk in a saucepan over high heat. Add quinoa to the milk and again bring it to a boil. Let it simmer for 15 minutes on low heat until milk is reduced.

2.   Stir in cinnamon and mix well. Cover and cook for 8 minutes until the milk is completely absorbed.

3.   Add blueberries and cook for 30 seconds. Serve and enjoy.

Nutrition

Calories: 271 Fat: 3.7g Carbs: 54g Protein: 6.5g   Fiber: 3.5g

Amaranth Porridge

Preparation Time: 5 minutes | **Cooking Time:** 30 minutes | **Servings:** 2

Ingredients:

o   2 cups of coconut milk

o   2 cups alkaline water

o   1 cup amaranth

o   2 tablespoons coconut oil

o   1 tablespoon ground cinnamon

Directions:

1. Mix milk with water in a medium saucepan. Bring the mixture to a boil. Stir in amaranth, then reduce the heat to low. Cook on a low simmer for 30 minutes with occasional stirring.
2. Turn off the heat, then stir in cinnamon and coconut oil. Serve warm.

Nutrition

Calories: 434 Fat: 35g Carbs: 27g Protein: 6.7g Fiber: 3.6g

Banana Barley Porridge

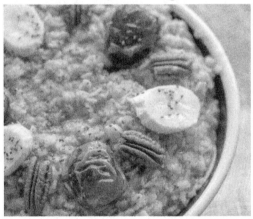

Preparation Time: 15 minutes | **Cooking Time**: 5 minutes | **Servings**: 2

Ingredients:

o   1 cup unsweetened coconut milk, divided

o   1 small banana, peeled and sliced

o   ½ cup barley

o   3 drops liquid stevia

o   ¼ cup coconuts, chopped

Directions:

1. Mix barley with half coconut milk and stevia in a bowl and mix well. Cover and refrigerate for about 6 hours.
2. Mix the barley mixture with coconut milk in a saucepan. Cook for 5 minutes on medium heat. Top with chopped coconuts and banana slices.
3. Serve.

Nutrition

Calories: 159 Fat: 8.4g Carbs: 19.8g Protein: 4.6g Fiber: 4.1g

Zucchini Muffins

Preparation Time: 10 minutes | **Cooking Time**: 25 minutes | **Servings**: 16

Ingredients:

o   1 tablespoon ground flaxseed

o   3 tablespoons alkaline water

o   ¼ cup walnut butter

o   3 small-medium over-ripe bananas

o   2 small zucchinis, grated

o   ½ cup of coconut milk

o   1 teaspoon vanilla extract

o   2 cups coconut flour

o   1 tablespoon baking powder

o   1 teaspoon cinnamon

o   ¼ teaspoon of sea salt

Directions:

1. Set your oven to 375 F, then grease a muffin tray with cooking spray. Mix flaxseed with water in a bowl.
2. Mash bananas in a glass bowl and stir in all the remaining **Ingredients**. Mix well and divide the mixture into the muffin tray—Bake for 25 minutes.
3. Serve.

Nutrition:

Calories: 127 Fat: 6.6g Carbs: 13g Protein: 0.7g Fiber: 0.7g

Millet Porridge

Preparation Time: 10 minutes | **Cooking Time**: 20 minutes | **Servings**: 2

Ingredients:

o   Pinch of sea salt

o   1 tablespoon coconuts, chopped finely

o   ½ cup unsweetened coconut milk

o   ½ cup millet, rinsed and drained

o   1½ cups alkaline water

o   3 drops liquid stevia

Directions:

1. Sauté millet in a non-stick skillet for 3 minutes. Stir in salt and water. Let it boil, then reduce the heat.

2. Cook for 15 minutes, then stirs in remaining **Ingredients**. Cook for another 4 minutes. Serve with chopped nuts on top.

Nutrition

Calories: 219 Fat: 4.5g Carbs: 38.2g Protein: 6.4g Fiber: 5g

Jackfruit Vegetable Fry

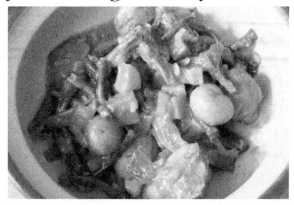

Preparation Time: 5 minutes | **Cooking Time**: 5 minutes | **Servings**: 6

Ingredients:

o   2 small onions, finely chopped

o   2 cups cherry tomatoes, finely chopped

o   1/8 teaspoon ground turmeric

o   1 tablespoon olive oil

o   2 red bell peppers, seeded and chopped

o   3 cups firm jackfruit, seeded and chopped

o   1/8 teaspoon cayenne pepper

o   2 tablespoons fresh basil leaves, chopped

o   Salt, to taste

Directions:

1.   Sauté onions and bell peppers in a greased skillet for 5 minutes. Stir in tomatoes and cook for 2 minutes.

2.   Add turmeric, salt, cayenne pepper, and jackfruit— Cook for 8 minutes. Garnish with basil leaves. Serve warm.

Nutrition

Calories: 236 Fat: 1.8g Carbs: 48.3g Protein: 7g

Zucchini Pancakes

Preparation Time: 15 minutes | **Cooking Time**: 8 minutes | **Servings**: 8

Ingredients:

o   12 tablespoons alkaline water

o   6 large zucchinis, grated

o   Sea salt, to taste

o   4 tablespoons ground Flax Seeds

o   2 teaspoons olive oil

o   2 jalapeño peppers, finely chopped

o   ½ cup scallions, finely chopped

Directions:

1.   Mix water plus flax seeds in a bowl and keep aside.

2.   Heat oil in a large non-stick skillet on medium heat and add zucchini, salt, and black pepper.

3.   Cook for about 3 minutes and transfer the zucchini into a large bowl. Stir in scallions and flaxseed mixture and thoroughly mix.

4.   Preheat a griddle and grease it lightly with cooking spray. Pour about ¼ of the zucchini mixture into preheated griddle and cook for about 3 minutes.

5.   Flip the side carefully and cook for about 2 more minutes. Repeat with the remaining mixture in batches and serve.

Nutrition

Calories: 71 Fat: 2.8g Carbs: 9.8g Protein: 3.7g   Fiber: 3.9g

Squash Hash

Preparation Time: 2 minutes | **Cooking Time**: 10 minutes | **Servings**: 2

Ingredients:

o   1 teaspoon onion powder

o   ½ cup onion, finely chopped

o   2 cups spaghetti squash

o   ½ teaspoon of sea salt

Directions:

1.   Squeeze any extra moisture from spaghetti squash using paper towels. Place the squash into a bowl, then add the onion powder, onion, and salt. Stir to combine.

2.   Spray a non-stick cooking skillet with cooking spray and place it over medium heat.

3.   Add the spaghetti squash to the pan. Cook the squash for 5 minutes, untouched. Using a spatula, flip the hash browns.

4.   Cook for an extra 5 minutes or up until the desired crispness is reached.

5. Serve and Enjoy!

Nutrition

Calories: 44 Fat: 0.6g Carbs: 9.7g Protein: 0.9g Fiber: 0.6g

Hemp Seed Porridge

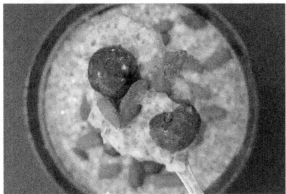

Preparation Time: 5 minutes

Cooking Time: 5 minutes

Servings: 6

Ingredients:

o   3 cups cooked hemp seed

o   1 packet Stevia

o   1 cup of coconut milk

Directions:

1. Mix the rice plus coconut milk in a saucepan over medium heat for 5 minutes.
2. Make sure to stir constantly. Remove, and mix in the stevia, then divide among 6 bowls. Serve and Enjoy!

Nutrition:

Calories: 236 Fat: 1.8g Carbs: 48.3g Protein: 7g Fiber: 0.6g

Veggie Medley

Preparation Time: 5 minutes | **Cooking Time**: 10 minutes | **Servings**: 2

Ingredients:

o   1 bell pepper, seeded, any color and sliced

o   juice of ½ a lime

o   2 tablespoons fresh cilantro

o   ½ teaspoon cumin

o   1 teaspoon of sea salt

o   1 jalapeno, chopped

o   ½ cup zucchini, sliced

o   1 cup cherry tomatoes, halved

o   ½ cup mushrooms, sliced

o   1 cup broccoli florets, cooked

o   1 sweet onion, chopped

Directions:

1. Grease a non-stick pan using a cooking spray and place it over medium heat.
2. Add the onion, broccoli, bell pepper, tomatoes, zucchini, mushrooms, and jalapeno. Cook for 7 minutes, or up until preferred doneness is reached. Stir occasionally.
3. Stir in the cumin, cilantro, and salt. Cook for 3 minutes while stirring. Remove pan from heat, then add the lime juice. Divide between serving plates, serve, and enjoy!

Nutrition:

Calories: 86 Fat: 0.07g Carbs: 17.4g Protein: 4.1g Fiber: 5.1g

Pumpkin Spice Quinoa

Preparation Time: 10 minutes | **Cooking Time**: 0 minutes | **Servings**: 2

Ingredients:

o   1 cup cooked quinoa

o   1 cup unsweetened coconut milk

o   1 large banana, mashed

o   1/4 cup pumpkin puree

o   1 teaspoon pumpkin spice

o   2 teaspoon chia seeds

Directions:

1. Mix all the Ingredients in a container.
2. Seal and shake well to mix. Refrigerate overnight.
3. Serve.

Nutrition:

Calories: 212 Fat: 11.9g Carbs: 31.7g Protein: 7.3g Fiber: 2g

Zucchini Home Fries

Preparation Time: 5 minutes | **Cooking Time**: 20 minutes | **Servings**: 2

Ingredients:

o   4 medium zucchinis

o   1 teaspoon onion powder

o   1 teaspoon of sea salt

o 1 red bell pepper, seeded, diced

o ½ sweet white onion, chopped

o ¼ cup vegetable broth

o ½ cup mushrooms, sliced

Directions:

1. In a medium-sized microwave-safe bowl, microwave the 4 zucchinis for about 4 minutes or until soft. Allow zucchinis to cool.

2. Add the broth into a large non-stick pan over medium heat, add the red bell pepper and onion.

3. Sauté your vegetables for 5 minutes.

4. While the vegetables are cooking, slice your zucchinis into quarters.

5. Add the mushrooms, onion powder, salt, and zucchinis to the pan. Cook your mixture for about 10 minutes or until the zucchinis are crisp.

6. Serve and Enjoy!

Nutrition:

Calories: 337 Fat: 0.8g Carbs: 74.8g Protein: 9.3g Fiber: 12.4g

Blackberry Pie

Preparation Time: 10 minutes | **Cooking Time**: 10 minutes | **Servings**: 4

Ingredients:

o 1 vanilla bean, cut lengthwise, deseeded

o ¼ teaspoon cinnamon

o 6 cups blackberry, sliced

o ¼ cup unsweetened coconut milk

o ½ cup orange juice, freshly squeezed

Directions:

1. Combine all your **Ingredients**.

2. In a medium-size skillet on medium-high heat, cook the fruit mixture. Cook the fruit mixture for 10 minutes.

3. Divide the fruit mixture among four serving dishes. Top with 1 tablespoon of coconut milk. Serve and Enjoy!

Nutrition

Calories: 109 Fat: 0.1g Carbs: 28.5g Protein: 0.2g Fiber: 4.5g

Banana Muffins

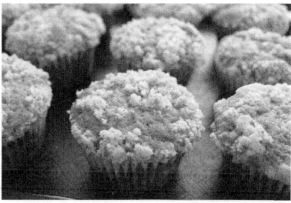

Preparation time: 25 Minutes | **Cooking time**: 20 minutes | **Servings**: 6

Ingredients

o ½ teaspoon salt

o 1 tablespoon vanilla extract

o 3 tablespoons ground flax seeds and 6-9 tablespoons water (egg substitute)

o 3 very ripe bananas, mashed

o ¼ cup oil

o 2 cups almond flour

o 1 tablespoon raw honey

o 1 teaspoon baking soda

Directions

1. Preheat your oven to 350 degrees F, and mix the flaxseed, honey, banana, vanilla and oil.

2. In a different bowl, mix the baking soda, almond flour and salt.

3. Gently add the dry Ingredients into the banana mixture.

4. Spoon the batter into a greased muffin tin and bake for about 15 minutes. Insert a toothpick to check if it is done.

Nutrition

Calories 140 Fat: 0.8g Carbs: 74.8g Protein: 9.3g

Flourless Banana Bread Muffins

Preparation time: 20 Minutes | **Cooking time**: 15 minutes | **Servings**: 9

Ingredients

o 3/4 cup almond flour/meal

o 2 tablespoons raw honey

o 1 teaspoon vanilla extract

o   1 tablespoon flaxseed plus 2 tablespoons water (combined)

o   ½ cup rolled oats

o   ½ teaspoon ground cinnamon

o   2 ripe medium bananas (200 g or a cup mashed)

o   2 tablespoons ground flaxseed

o   ¼ cup almond butter

o   ½ teaspoon baking soda

Directions

1. Preheat your oven to 375 degrees F and spray 9 cavities of your muffin tin with cooking spray. Place aside.
2. Toss all Ingredients into your blender and run on high until the oats are broken down and the batter turns creamy and smooth.
3. Pour the batter into the muffin tins; fill them about 3/4 full.
4. Bake for about 10 to 12 minutes until the top of the muffins is set. Insert toothpick to check for doneness.
5. Let the muffins cool approximately for 10 minutes before you remove them. The muffins can keep in an airtight container for 10 days.

Nutrition

Calories: 133 Fat: 0.8g Carbs: 44.8g Protein: 9.3g

Super Seed Spelt Pancakes

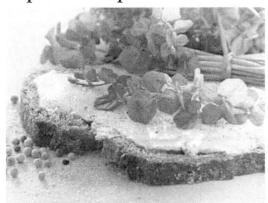

Preparation time: 15 Minutes | **Cooking time**: 10 minutes | **Servings**: 4

Ingredients

o   42g flax seeds

o   ½ teaspoon stevia extract

o   37.5g sesame seeds

o   ¼ teaspoon fine sea salt

o   80g chia seeds

o   164g buckwheat groats

o   1 ½ teaspoons ground cinnamon

o   ½ teaspoon baking powder

o   30g pumpkin seeds

o   2 tablespoons almond milk

o   1 teaspoon coconut oil

o   1 teaspoon baking soda

Directions

1. Grind the pumpkin seeds, sesame seeds, flax seeds, chia seeds and buckwheat groats into flour and keep ¼ of the seed flour for later use (not for this recipe).
2. Add 2 cups of the seed flour to a medium bowl.
3. Add in the rest of the Ingredients but not the coconut oil. Pour in more milk if needed to attain the right consistency.
4. Add coconut oil to a non-stick pan and place over heat.
5. Once heated, pour thin layers of the batter and flip once you see bubbles form on top.
6. Cook until all the batter is used up.

Nutrition

Calories: 110 Fat: 0.8g Carbs: 74.8g Protein: 9.3g

Scrambled Tofu

Preparation time: 10 Minutes | **Cooking time**: 15 minutes | **Servings**: 1

Ingredients

o   3 cloves

o   1 onion

o   1/2 teaspoon of turmeric

o   Salt for taste

o   50g firm tofu

o   1/2 teaspoon of paprika

o   1 handful baby spinach

o   3 tomatoes

o   1/2 cup of yeast

o   1/2 teaspoon of cumin

Directions

1. Mince the garlic and dice up the onion.
2. Toss the onions into a pan and let them cook over medium heat for about 7 minutes. Add in the garlic and cook for 1 minute.

3. Toss in the tofu and tomatoes and cook for 10 more minutes. Add in some water, cumin and paprika and stir well. Continue cooking.

4. When the dish is about to cook, add in spinach, stir and once wilted, turn off the heat and serve.

Nutrition

Calories: 121 Fat: 6g Protein: 3g Carbs: 3g

Ginger-Maple Yam Casserole

Preparation time: 10 minutes | **Cooking time**: 40 minutes | **Servings**: 4

Ingredients:

o 2 yams, peeled and cut into ½-inch chunks

o ¼ cup fresh ginger, peeled and grated

o 2 tbsp. avocado oil

o 2 tbsp. pure maple syrup

o 4 tsp. cardamom

o A pinch of sea salt

Directions:

1. Preheat the oven to 375F.

2. In a casserole dish, combine the yams, ginger, oil, maple syrup, cardamom, and salt. Mix well.

3. Cover and bake for 40 minutes.

4. Serve.

Nutrition

Calories: 144 Fat: 7g Carbohydrates: 20g

Ginger-Sesame Quinoa with Vegetables

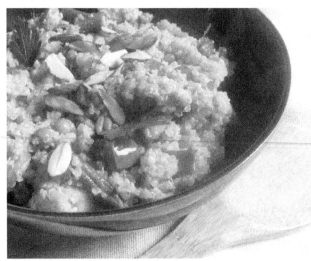

Preparation time: 10 minutes | **Cooking time**: 30 minutes | **Servings**: 4

Ingredients:

o 1 cup quinoa

o 2 cups low-sodium vegetable stock

o 1 tbsp. tahini

o 4 tsp. fresh ginger, peeled and minced

o A pinch of sea salt, plus more for seasoning

o 2 carrots, finely chopped

o 1 red bell pepper, finely chopped

o 1 cup snow peas, stringed and halved

o 2 tsp. sesame seeds

o Sesame oil, for garnish

Directions:

1. Preheat the oven to 325F.

2. In a casserole dish, combine the stock, quinoa, tahini, ginger, and salt. Mix.

3. Add in the pepper, carrots, and snow peas. Mix well.

4. Cover and bake for 30 minutes.

5. Top with sesame seeds and a drizzle of sesame oil.

6. Adjust seasoning with salt and serve.

Nutrition

Calories: 261 Fat: 3g Carbohydrates: 46g Protein: 10g

Vegetarian Pie

Preparation time: 20 minutes | **Cooking time**: 1 hour 20 minutes | **Servings**: 8

Ingredients:

for Topping

o 5 cups water

o 1¼ cups yellow cornmeal

For Filing

o 1 tbsp. extra-virgin olive oil

o 1 large onion, chopped

o 1 medium red bell pepper, seeded and chopped

o 2 garlic cloves, minced

o 1 tsp. dried oregano, crushed

o 2 tsp. chili powder

o 2 cups fresh tomatoes, chopped

o 2½ cups Cooked pinto beans

o 2 cups boiled corn kernels

Directions:

1. Preheat the oven to 375 F. Lightly grease a shallow baking dish.

2. In a pan, add the water over medium-high heat and bring to a boil.

3. Slowly, add the cornmeal, stirring continuously.

4. Reduce the heat to low and Cooking covered for about 20 minutes, stirring occasionally.

5. Meanwhile, Prepare the filling. In a large skillet, heat the oil over medium heat and sauté the onion and bell pepper for about 3-4 minutes.

6. Add the garlic, oregano, and spices and sauté for about 1 minute

7. Add the remaining Ingredients and stir to combine.

8. Reduce the heat to low and simmer for about 10-15 minutes, stirring occasionally.

9. Remove from the heat.

10. Place half of the Cooked cornmeal into the Prepared baking dish evenly.

11. Place the filling mixture over the cornmeal evenly.

12. Place the remaining cornmeal over the filling mixture evenly.

13. Bake for 45-50 minutes or until the top becomes golden brown.

14. Remove the pie from the oven and set it aside for about 5 minutes before serving.

Nutrition

Calories: 350 Fat: 3.9g Carb: 58.2g Protein: 16.8g

Red Thai Vegetable Curry

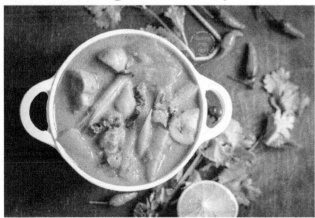

Preparation time: 10 minutes | **Cooking time**: 15 minutes | **Servings**: 4

Ingredients:

o   2 cups vegetable stock

o   1 sweet potato, rinsed and chopped

o   1 head broccoli, rinsed and chopped

o   1 eggplant, rinsed and chopped

o   1 zucchini, rinsed and chopped

o   1 red bell pepper, rinsed and chopped

o   1½ cups canned, full-fat coconut milk

o   1 tablespoon red Thai curry paste

o   2 kaffir lime leaves

o   1 (1-inch) piece fresh ginger, peeled and grated

o   Himalayan pink salt

o   Freshly ground black pepper

o   2 tablespoons coconut aminos

o   Juice of 1 lime

Directions:

1. In a large pot over high heat, bring the vegetable stock to a boil. Add the sweet potato, broccoli, eggplant, zucchini, red bell pepper, coconut milk, curry paste, lime leaves, and ginger. Reduce the heat to low and cook for 10 minutes, stirring frequently.

2. Taste and season with salt and pepper. Simmer for 5 minutes more.

3. Remove the pot from the heat, stir in the coconut aminos and lime juice, and serve.

Nutrition:

Calories: 300 Total fat: 19g Total carbohydrates: 23g Fiber: 9g Sugar: 11g Protein: 7g

Thick Alkaline Minestrone

Preparation time: 10 minutes | **Cooking time**: 15 minutes | **Servings**: 2

Ingredients:

o   1 tablespoon coconut oil

o   ¼ onion, rinsed and diced

o   2 garlic cloves, minced

o   ½ cup sweet potato, scrubbed and cubed

o   ½ cup zucchini, rinsed and cubed

o   ½ cup eggplant, rinsed and cubed

o   ½ cup carrot, rinsed and diced

o   ½ cup canned beans, such as white, navy, or kidney beans, rinsed and drained

o   1 cup tomato juice

o   ½ cup vegetable stock

o   Handful fresh basil leaves, rinsed

o   Himalayan pink salt

o   Freshly ground black pepper

Directions:

1. In a large pot over medium-high heat, heat the coconut oil. Add the onion, garlic, sweet potato, zucchini, eggplant, and carrot. Sauté for 3 minutes.
2. Stir in the beans, tomato juice, and vegetable stock. Bring to a boil. Reduce the heat to simmer and cook for 10 minutes.
3. Stir in the basil, season with salt and pepper, and serve.

Nutrition:

Calories: 168 Total fat: 7g Total carbohydrates: 25g Fiber: 6g Sugar: 11g Protein: 4g

Sprouted Buckwheat Crepes

Preparation time: 15 Minutes | **Cooking time**: 10 minutes | **Servings**: 4

Ingredients

o   1 tablespoon pure 100% vanilla extract
o   ¾ cup pure water
o   1 cup buckwheat groats- soaked overnight
o   1 tablespoon chia seeds

Directions

1. Rinse buckwheat thoroughly and soak it in 1:2 parts water overnight.
2. Rinse then drain well the following morning.
3. Add all your **Ingredients** to a blender and process until smooth.
4. Add coconut oil to a nonstick pan over high medium heat and pour in a thin layer to the center of your pan. Swirl the pan to make sure the batter spreads out- the texture should be thick enough to hold the shape for flipping.
5. Once the top is not liquid, flip and cook the other side until browned.
6. Do this with the rest of the batter.
7. Serve with some sprouted nut butter, fresh lemon juice, hemp seeds or whatever you like.

Nutrition

Calories: 202 Fat: 0.8g Carbs: 74.8g Protein: 9.3g

Butternut Squash, Apple Casserole with Drizzle

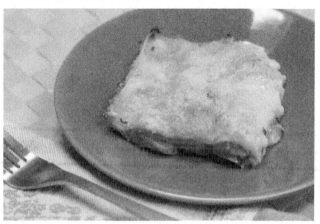

Preparation time: 10 minutes | **Cooking time**: 30 minutes | **Servings**: 4

Ingredients:

o   1 butternut squash, peeled, seeded, and cut into ½-inch chunks
o   2 Granny Smith apples, cored and cut into ½-inch chunks
o   1 white onion, cut into ½-inch chunks
o   4 garlic cloves, coarsely chopped
o   ½ tbsp. avocado oil
o   ½ tbsp. pure maple syrup
o   2 tsp. ground cinnamon
o   ½ tsp. chili powder
o   A pinch of sea salt
o   A pinch of freshly ground black pepper

Directions:

1. Preheat the oven to 375F.
2. In a large casserole dish, combine the apples, squash, onion, garlic, oil, syrup, cinnamon, chili powder, salt, and pepper. Mix well.
3. Cover and bake for 30 minutes.
4. Serve.

Nutrition:

Calories: 123 Fat: 2g Carb: 28g Protein: 2g

Breakfast Salad

Preparation time: 10 Minutes | **Cooking time**: 15 minutes | **Servings**: 2

Ingredients

o   1/2 pack of firm tofu
o   ½ a red onion

- o   2 spelt tortillas
- o   1 avocado
- o   4 handfuls of baby spinach
- o   1 handful of almonds
- o   2 tomatoes
- o   1 pink grapefruit
- o   1/2 lemon

Directions

1. Heat up the tortillas in an oven and once warm, bake for 8 to 10 minutes in the oven.
2. Chop up the onions, tomatoes and tofu and combine this. Put in the fridge and let it cool.
3. Now chop up the almonds, avocado and grapefruit. Mix everything well and place nicely around the bowl you had put in the fridge.
4. Squeeze a lemon on top all over the salad and enjoy!

Nutrition

Calories: 80 Total fat: 12g Total carbohydrates: 32g
Fiber: 3g Sugar: 15g Protein: 9g

Scrambled Tofu and Tomato

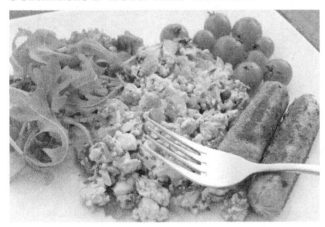

Preparation time: 15 Minutes | **Cooking time**: 15 minutes | **Servings**: 2

Ingredients

- o   1 tablespoon coconut oil
- o   A little coriander/cilantro
- o   285g regular firm tofu
- o   2 big handfuls of baby spinach
- o   1/2 brown onion (or red if you fancy)
- o   1 handful of arugula/rocket
- o   Freshly ground black pepper
- o   2 tomatoes
- o   Himalayan/Sea salt
- o   Pinch of turmeric
- o   A little basil
- o   ½ small red pepper
- o   A pinch of cayenne pepper

Directions

1. Use your hands to scramble the tofu into a bowl then chop and fry the onion quickly in a pan. Dice the peppers and do the same thing.
2. Dice the tomatoes and throw them into the pan. Toss in a pinch of turmeric, and add the spinach. Add salt and grind in the pepper. Cook until the tofu is warm and cooked.
3. Throw in basil leaves, coriander, the rocket just when the meal is about to be done. Serve with a pinch of some hot cayenne pepper.
4. You can serve on some toasted sprouted bread and some baby spinach.

Nutrition:

Calories: 144 Fat: 0.8g Carbs: 74.8g Protein: 9.3g

Lunch recipes

Tomato Soup

Preparation time: 15 minutes | **Cooking time**: 15 minutes | **Servings**: 4

Ingredients:

o 2 teaspoons avocado oil

o 1 medium white onion, chopped

o 3 garlic cloves, minced

o 7 cups fresh plum tomatoes, chopped

o ½ cup fresh sweet basil, chopped

o Sea salt, as needed

o ¼ teaspoon cayenne powder

Directions:

1. In a pan, heat the oil over medium heat and sauté the onion and garlic for about 5–6 minutes.
2. Add the tomatoes and cook for about 6–8 minutes, crushing with the back of spoon occasionally.
3. Stir in the basil, salt, and cayenne powder and remove from the heat.
4. With a hand blender, puree the soup mixture until smooth.
5. Serve immediately.

Nutrition:

Calories 75 Total Fat 1 g Saturated Fat 0.2 g Cholesterol 0 mg Sodium 56 mg Total Carbs 15.8 g Fiber 4.6 g Sugar 9.5 g Protein 3.5 g

Mushroom Soup

Preparation time: 15 minutes | **Cooking time**: 25 minutes | **Servings**: 4

Ingredients

o 2 teaspoons avocado oil

o 1¼ cups fresh Portobello mushrooms, sliced

o 1¼ cups fresh button mushrooms, sliced

o ½ cup white onion, chopped

o 1 garlic clove, crushed

o ½ teaspoon dried thyme

o Sea salt and cayenne powder, as needed

o 1¾ cups unsweetened coconut milk

o 1½ cups spring water

Directions:

1. In a soup pan, heat the avocado oil over medium-high heat and cook the mushrooms, onions, garlic, thyme, salt, and black pepper for about 5–6 minutes.
2. Add in the coconut milk and water and bring to a boil.
3. Now, adjust the heat to medium-low and simmer for about 10–15 minutes, stirring occasionally.
4. Serve hot.

Nutrition

Calories 177 Total Fat 14.9 g Saturated Fat 13.2 g Cholesterol 0 mg Sodium 75 mg Total Carbs 5.9g Fiber 0.9 g   Sugar 4 g Protein 2.9 g

Mixed Greens Soup

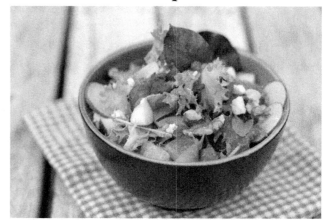

Preparation time: 15 minutes | **Cooking time**: 5 minutes | **Servings**: 3

Ingredients:

o 2 cups fresh kale, tough ribs removed and chopped

o 2 cups fresh watercress

o 2 cups dandelion greens

o 2 garlic cloves, peeled

o 2 cups spring water

o 1 cup unsweetened coconut milk

o 1 tablespoon fresh key lime juice

o ½ teaspoon cayenne powder

o Sea salt, as needed

Directions:

1. Place all soup ingredients in a high-powered blender and pulse on high speed until smooth.

2. Transfer the soup into a pan over medium heat and cook for about 3–5 minutes or until heated through.

3. Serve hot.

Nutrition

Calories 168 Total Fat 11.4 g Saturated Fat 10.1 g Cholesterol 0 mg Sodium 137 mg Total Carbs11g Fiber 2.4 g Sugar 2.4 g Protein 4.2 g

Squash & Apple Soup

Preparation time: 15 minutes | **Cooking time:** 45 minutes | **Servings:** 4

Ingredients

o   2 tablespoon avocado oil

o   1 cup white onion, chopped

o   2 garlic cloves, minced

o   1 teaspoon dried thyme

o   3 cups butternut squash, peeled and cubed

o   2 apples, cored and chopped

o   4 cups spring water

o   Sea salt, as needed

Directions:

1. In a soup pan, heat avocado oil over medium heat and sauté the onion for about 5 minutes.

2. Add the garlic and thyme and sauté for about 1 minute.

3. Add the squash and apple and ginger and cook for about 1–2 minutes.

4. Stir in the water and bring to a boil.

5. Now, adjust the heat to low and simmer covered for about 30 minutes.

6. Stir in the salt and remove from the heat.

7. With a hand blender, puree the soup mixture until smooth.

8. Serve immediately.

Nutrition

Calories 129 Total Fat 1.3 g Saturated Fat 0.2 g Cholesterol 0 mg Sodium 46 mg Total Carbs 31.4 g Fiber 5.9 g Sugar 15.2 g Protein 1.9 g

Chickpeas & Squash Stew

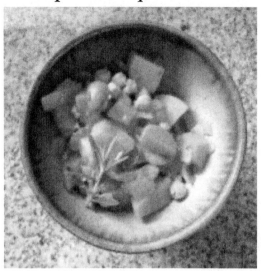

Preparation time: 15 minutes | **Cooking time:** 1¼ hours | **Servings:** 4

Ingredients:

o   2 tablespoons avocado oil

o   1 large white onion, chopped

o   4 garlic cloves, minced

o   ½ tablespoon cayenne powder

o   4 large plum tomatoes, seeded and chopped finely

o   1 pound butternut squash; peeled, seeded, and chopped

o   1½ cups spring water

o   1 cup cooked chickpeas

o   2 tablespoons fresh key lime juice

o   Sea salt, as needed

o   2 tablespoons fresh parsley, chopped

Directions:

1. In a soup pan, heat the avocado oil over medium heat and sauté the onion for about 4–6 minutes.

2. Add the garlic and cayenne powder and sauté for about 1 minute.

3. Add the tomatoes and cook for about 2–3 minutes.

4. Add the squash and water and bring to a boil.

5. Now, adjust the heat to low and simmer, covered for about 50 minutes.

6. Add the chickpeas and cook for about 10 minutes.

7. Stir in lime juice and salt and remove from heat.

8. Serve hot with the garnishing of parsley.

Nutrition

Calories 150 Total Fat 1.8 g Saturated Fat 0.3 g
Cholesterol 0 mg Sodium 188 mg Total Carbs 21.5g

Chickpeas & Kale Stew

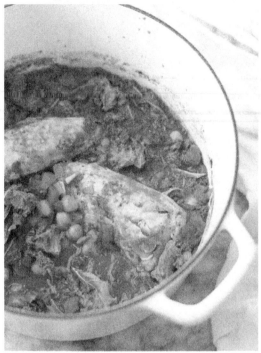

Preparation time: 15 minutes | **Cooking time:** 30 minutes | **Servings:** 4

Ingredients:

o   1 tablespoon avocado oil

o   1 large onion, chopped

o   2 garlic cloves, minced

o   3 cups cherry tomatoes, chopped finely

o   2 cups spring water

o   2 cups cooked chickpeas

o   2 cups fresh kale, tough ribs removed and chopped

o   1 tablespoon fresh key lime juice

o   Sea salt, as needed

o   ¼ teaspoon cayenne powder

Directions:

1.   In a soup pan, heat avocado oil over medium heat and sauté the onion for about 6 minutes.

2.   Stir in the garlic and sauté for about 1 minute.

3.   Add the tomatoes and cook for about 2–3 minutes.

4.   Add the water and bring to a boil.

5.   Now, adjust the heat to low and simmer for about 10 minutes.

6.   Stir in the chickpeas and simmer for about 5 minutes.

7.   Stir in the spinach and simmer for 3–4 minutes more.

8.   Stir in the lime juice and seasoning and remove from the heat.

9.   Serve hot.

Nutrition:

Calories 206 Total Fat 2.1 g Saturated Fat 0.3 g
Cholesterol 0 mg Sodium 421 mg Total Carbs 40.1g
Fiber 8.4 g Sugar 5.2 g Protein 8.7 g

Chickpeas & Veggie Stew

Preparation time: 20 minutes | **Cooking time:** 1 hour 5 minutes | **Servings:** 6

Ingredients:

o   3 cups portabella mushrooms, chopped

o   4 cups spring water

o   1 cup cooked chickpeas

o   1 cup fresh kale, tough ribs removed and chopped

o   1 cup white onion, chopped

o   1 cup green bell peppers, seeded and chopped

o   ½ cup butternut squash; peeled, seeded, and chopped

o   2 plum tomatoes, chopped

o   2 tablespoons grapeseed oil

o   1 teaspoon dried oregano

o   1 teaspoon dried basil

o   ½ teaspoon dried thyme

o   2 teaspoons onion powder

o   1 teaspoon cayenne powder

o   ½ teaspoon ginger powder

o   Sea salt, as needed

Directions:

1.   In a soup pan, add all ingredients over high heat and bring to a rolling boil.

2.   Now, adjust the heat to low and simmer, covered for about 1 hour, stirring occasionally.

3.   Serve hot.

Nutrition:

Calories 201 Total Fat 6.9 g Saturated Fat 0.7 g
Cholesterol 0 mg Sodium 49 mg Total Carbs 28.6 g
Fiber 7.6 g Sugar 7.4 g Protein 8.8 g

Quinoa & Veggie Stew

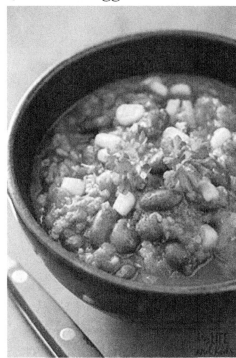

Preparation time: 15 minutes | **Cooking time:** 1 hour
Servings: 4 |
Ingredients:

o   2 tablespoons grapeseed oil

o   1 large onion, chopped

o   Sea salt, as needed

o   2 cups butternut squash, peeled and cubed

o   3 garlic cloves, minced

o   1 teaspoon ground cumin

o   1 teaspoon cayenne powder

o   2½ cups plum tomatoes, chopped finely

o   ½ cup dry quinoa, rinsed

o   3 cups spring water

o   3 cups fresh kale, tough ribs removed and chopped

o   1 tablespoon fresh key lime juice

Directions:

1. In a soup pan, heat the grapeseed oil over medium heat and cook the onion with few pinches of salt for about 4–5 minutes, stirring occasionally.

2. Add the butternut squash and cook for about 3–4 minutes.

3. Stir in the garlic and spices and cook for about 1 minute.

4. Stir in the tomatoes, quinoa, and water and bring to a boil.

5. Now, adjust the heat to low and simmer, covered for about 35 minutes.

6. Stir in the kale and cook for about 10 minutes.

Nutrition:
Calories 237 Total Fat 8.6 g Saturated Fat 0.9 g
Cholesterol 0 mg Sodium 73 mg Total Carbs 36.2 g
Fiber 6 g Sugar 6.2 g Protein 6.9 g

Mango & Apple Sauce

Preparation time: 10 minutes | **Cooking time:** 0 minutes | **Servings:** 6
Ingredients:

o   1 cup mango; peeled, pitted, and chopped

o   2 large apples; peeled, cored, and chopped

o   3–4 tablespoons fresh key lime juice

o   2 tablespoons agave nectar

o   ½ cup fresh orange juice

Directions:

1. Add all the sauce ingredients in a high-powered blender and pulse on high speed until smooth.

2. Serve immediately.

Nutrition:
Calories 85 Total Fat 0.3 g Saturated Fat 0 g
Cholesterol 0 mg Sodium 1 mg Total Carbs 22 g
Fiber 2.6 g Sugar 18.2 g Protein 0.6 g

Tomato Sauce

Preparation time: 15 minutes | **Cooking time:** 50 minutes | **Servings:** 24
Ingredients:

o   18 plum tomatoes, halved

o   ½ of red bell pepper, seeded and halved

o   ½ of red onion, halved

o   ½ of sweet onion, halved

o   1 medium shallot, halved

o   2 tablespoons grapeseed oil

o   3 teaspoons dried basil, divided

o   3 teaspoons sea salt

o   1 tablespoon agave nectar

o   2 teaspoons dried oregano

o   2 teaspoons onion powder

o   1/8 teaspoon cayenne powder

Directions:

1. Preheat your oven to 400°F.
2. Line a baking sheet with parchment paper.
3. In a bowl, add tomatoes, bell pepper, onions, shallot, oil, 1 teaspoon of basil, and 1 teaspoon of salt and toss to coat well.
4. Arrange the vegetables onto the prepared baking sheet, cut side down.
5. Roast for about 30 minutes, flipping the vegetables once halfway through.
6. Remove the baking sheet from oven and set aside to cool slightly.
7. In a high-powered blender, add the roasted vegetables and pulse on high speed until smooth.
8. In a pan, add the pureed vegetables and remaining ingredients over low heat and simmer for about 20 minutes.
9. Remove from the heat and set aside to cool completely before serving.

Nutrition:

Calories 33 Total Fat 1.3 g Saturated Fat 0.1 g Cholesterol 0 mg Sodium 239 mg Total Carbs 5.3 g Fiber .4 g Sugar 3.4 g Protein 0.9 g

Artichoke Sauce Ala Quinoa Pasta

Preparation Time: 15 minutes | **Cooking Time:** 0 minute | **Servings:** 4

Ingredients:

o 7 ounce or 200g spelled pasta
o 8 ounce or 220g of frozen artichoke
o 5 ounces of fresh tomatoes
o 1 medium sized onion
o 1 clove of garlic
o 1 ounce of pine nuts
o 1 teaspoon of yeast free vegetable stock
o 3 tablespoons of fresh basil
o ½ a teaspoon of yeast free vegetable stock
o 3 tablespoons of fresh basil
o ½ a teaspoon of organic sea salt
o 1 pinch of cayenne pepper
o 2 tablespoon of cold pressed extra virgin olive oil

Directions:

1. Prepare your Artichokes by cooking them gently until they show a tender texture
2. Cook the pasta to Al Dente following the instructions on your packet

3. Take out your tomatoes and cut them up into cubes
4. Chop up the onions, garlic, and basil into bite sized portions
5. Take a pan and add 2 tablespoons of olive oil over medium heat
6. Add pine nuts, garlic, and onion and stir them for a few minutes
7. Take another bowl and add ½ a cup of water and dissolve yeast free veggie stock
8. Add the mixture to the pan. Simmer it over low heat and keep stirring it for 2 minutes
9. Once done, add basil and season with cayenne pepper and salt
10. Pour the sauce over your pasta. Serve!

Nutrition:

Calories 286 Fats 13g   Carbs 26g Fiber 3g

The Mysterious Alkaline Veggies and Rice

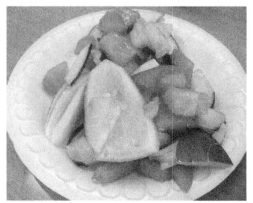

Preparation Time: 10 minutes | **Cooking Time:** 5 minutes | **Servings:** 4

Ingredients:

o 1 cup of wild rice
o 1 cup of Pak Choi
o 1 cup of Broccoli
o 1 cup of Young Beans
o 2 cups of Carrots
o 1 cup of bean sprout
o ½ a cup of vegetable broth
o 1 piece of chili
o 1 fresh juice of lime
o Cilantro as needed
o Basil as required

o Seas Salt as required

Directions:

1. Chop up the Pak Choi, carrots, beans, bean sprouts, and broccoli
2. Add them to a pan and pour vegetable broth
3. Steam fries the mixture until they are fully cooked and are a bit crunchy
4. Take a mortar and pestle and add cilantro and chopped up chili
5. Pour lime juice and mix well to prepare the dressing
6. Take a serving platter add rice, add the prepped vegetables
7. Serve by pouring the dressing over them!

Nutrition:

Calories 200 Fats 2g Carbs 33g Fiber 2g

Beautifully Curried Eggplant

Preparation Time: 5 minutes | **Cooking Time:** 5 minutes | **Servings:** 2

Ingredients:

o 1 piece of roasted eggplant (make sure to remove the contents from the shell and reserve juice from about 1 lemon)
o 1 teaspoon of sea salt
o 1 teaspoon of curry powder
o Water as required
o Cooked quinoa required for serving

Directions:

1. Take a food processor and add eggplant, lemon juice, sesame oil, salt, curry powder and blend the whole mixture well. Take a small sized saucepan and place it over medium heat
2. Add the eggplant mix to your saucepan and gently warm it for about 5 minutes. Add water to thin it if required. Serve the curried eggplants over some delicious quinoa!

Nutrition

Calories 81 Fats 2.8g Carbs 14g Fiber 8g Protein 8g

Coconut Milk and Glazing Stir Fried Tofu

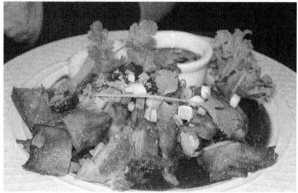

Preparation Time: 10 minutes | **Cooking Time:** 5 minutes | **Servings:** 4

Ingredients:

o 1 pound of firm tofu
o 3 medium sized Zucchinis
o 3 pieces of tomatoes
o 1 piece of red bell pepper
o 1 piece of green bell pepper
o ½ a pound of green beans
o 1 to 1 and a ½ cup of fresh coconut milk
o 2 tablespoon of cold pressed extra virgin olive oil
o Sea salt as needed
o Pepper as needed
o ½ a tablespoon of curry powder
o ¼ tablespoon of ginger
o Fresh assorted selection of Herbs

Directions:

1. Dice your tofu. Chop up your zucchinis. Chop up the bell peppers, tomatoes, beans into small portions. Take a pan and place it over medium heat, add oil and heat it up
2. Add tofu and fry them for about 2-3 minutes. Add pepper bell, beans, zucchini and stir fry for 2-3 minutes. Add tomatoes and coconut milk and stir well and cook for a while
3. Season with some ginger, salt, pepper, curry powder, and herbs. Serve with some wild rice or soba noodles

Nutrition

Calories 210 Fats 17g Carbs 8g Fiber 3g Protein 12g

Culturally Diverse Pumpkin Potato Patties

Preparation Time: 10 minutes | **Cooking Time:** 5 minutes | **Servings:** 2

Ingredients:

o   1 pound of 450g pumpkin

o   1 pound of 450g potatoes

o   ounce of soy 75g soy flour

o   4 tablespoons of water

o   3 tablespoons of chopped up parsley

o   Sea salt as needed

o   Organic salt as needed

o   Just a pinch of pepper

o   Cold Pressed Extra virgin olive oil

Directions:

1.   Peel the skin of your pumpkin and potatoes. Take a grater and grate both into chunky pieces. Take a bowl and add 2 tablespoons of soy flour and 4 tablespoons of water

2.   Take another bowl and add your grated potatoes and pumpkin alongside soy flour. Add flour to the mix and mix them well.

3.   Season with a bit of salt, parsley, and pepper. Take a pan and place it over medium heat. Add oil and heat it up. Prepare patties from the mixture and fry them in hot oil for about 2-3 minutes until they are brown

Nutrition

Calories 375 Fats 16g Carbs 46g Fiber 7g

Veggie Balls in Tomato Sauce

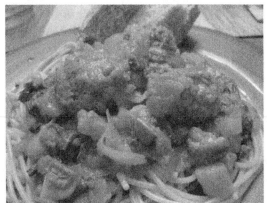

Preparation Time: 20 minutes | **Cooking Time:** 15 minutes | **Servings:** 8

Ingredients:

o   1½ cups cooked chickpeas

o   2 cups fresh button mushrooms

o   ½ cup onions, chopped

o   ¼ cup green bell peppers, seeded and chopped

o   2 teaspoons oregano

o   2 teaspoons fresh basil

o   1 teaspoon savory

o   1 teaspoon dried sage

o   1 teaspoon dried dill

o   1 tablespoon onion powder

o   ½ teaspoon cayenne powder

o   ½ teaspoon ginger powder

o   Sea salt, as required

o   ½-1 cup chickpea flour

o   6 cups homemade tomato sauce

o   2 tablespoons grapeseed oil

Directions:

1.   In a food processor, add the chickpeas, veggies, herbs and spices and pulse until well combined. Transfer the mixture into a large bowl with flour and mix until well combined. Make desired-sized balls from the mixture.

2.   Cook the oil over medium-high heat and let the balls cook in 2 batches for about 4-5 minutes or until golden brown from all sides.

3.   In a large pan, add the tomato sauce and veggie balls over medium heat and simmer for about 5 minutes. Serve hot.

Nutrition:

Calories 159 Total Fat 4.8g Protein 7.2g Carbs 23.9g Fiber 6g

Veggie Kabobs

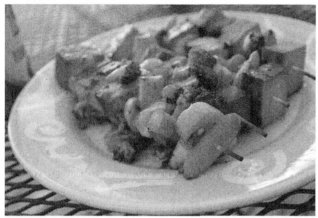

Preparation Time: 20 minutes | **Cooking Time:** 10 minutes | **Serves:** 4

Ingredients:

For Marinade

o   2 garlic cloves, minced

o   2 teaspoons fresh basil, minced

o   2 teaspoons fresh oregano, minced

o   ½ teaspoon cayenne powder

o   Sea salt, as required

o   2 tablespoons fresh key lime juice

o   2 tablespoons avocado oil

For Veggies

o   2 large zucchinis, cut into thick slices

o   8 large button mushrooms, quartered

o   1 yellow bell pepper, seeded and cubed

o   1 red bell pepper, seeded and cubed

Directions:

For marinade:

1.   Mix all the ingredients in a bowl. Mix in the vegetables and toss it well for evenly coat. Cover and refrigerate to marinate for at least 6-8 hours.

2.   Preheat the grill to medium-high heat. Generously, grease the grill grate. Remove the vegetables from the bowl and thread onto pre-soaked wooden skewers.

3.   Grill for about 8-10 minutes or until done completely, flipping occasionally.

Nutrition

Calories 122 Total Fat 7.8g Protein 4,3g Carbs 12.7g Fiber 3.5g

Spelt Spaghetti

Preparation Time: 10 minutes | **Cooking Time:** 20 minutes | **Servings:** 2-3

Ingredients:

o   1 – 8 oz. box of Spelt Spaghetti (Nature's Legacy makes a product that is only made from spelt and water.)

Directions:

1.   Boil 2 quarts of water in pot. Slowly add in the spelt spaghetti.

2.   Cook for 10 minutes, stirring occasionally. Don't overcook. Drain and plate.

Nutrition :

Calories 87 Protein 6.8 g Fiber 1.5g Protein 2g

Butternut Squash Plum Tomato Spaghetti Sauce

Preparation Time: 5 minutes | **Cooking Time:** 20 minutes | **Servings:** 4

Ingredients:

o   ½ butternut squash

o   ¼ plum tomato (chopped)

o   1 cup water

o   Spices: dash of cayenne pepper, onion, basil, bay leaf, oregano, thyme, savory, coriander, and salt

Directions:

1.   Add butternut squash cubes to pot, cover with water and boil until squash becomes tender. Remove squash from water.

2.   Add squash, tomato, and spices to a blender and blend, slowly add water until you reach desired consistency. Add to a container, let cool, and refrigerate.

Nutrition

Calories 105 Protein 21g Fiber 12g Protein 6g

Zucchini Turnip Soup

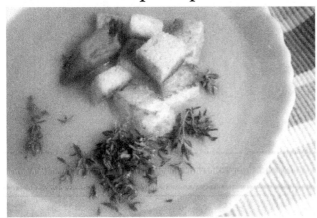

Preparation Time: 10 minutes | **Cooking Time:** 30 minutes | **Servings:** 4

Ingredients:

o 1 tablespoon coconut oil
o 2 cups yellow onion, chopped
o 2 cloves chive, minced
o 1 tablespoon fresh ginger, minced
o 2 tablespoons red curry paste
o 4 cups low-sodium vegetable broth
o 3 cups diced zucchinis, peeled
o 3 cups turnips, peeled and diced
o Celtic sea salt, iodine free, to taste
o Freshly ground black pepper to taste
o ¼ teaspoon cayenne pepper

Directions:

1. Sauté chive, onion, and ginger in a greased pan for 5 to 6 minutes. Stir in curry paste and broth.
2. Mix well then add zucchinis, salt, and turnips. Boil the soup on high heat. Cover the pot. Cook for 15 to 20 minutes. Blend this soup in a blender in batches until smooth.
3. Adjust seasoning with salt and pepper. Divide the soup into the serving bowl.
4. Serve warm.

Nutrition

Calories 338 Fat 3.8g Carbs 58.3g Protein 15.4g Fiber 2.4g

Quinoa Vegetable Soup

Preparation Time: 10 minutes | **Cooking Time:** 45 minutes | **Servings:** 4

Ingredients:

o 3 tablespoons coconut oil
o 1 medium yellow or white onion, chopped
o 3 zucchinis, peeled and chopped
o 2 celery stalks, chopped
o 1 cup zucchini or any seasonal vegetable
o 6 chive stalks, minced
o dried thyme, ½ teaspoon
o diced tomatoes, 28 oz., drained
o 1 cup quinoa, rinsed and drained
o vegetable broth, 4 cups
o alkaline water, 2 cups
o Celtic sea salt, 1 teaspoon, iodine free
o 2 bay leaves
o Pinch red pepper flakes
o Freshly ground black pepper, to taste
o Seville orange juice, 1 teaspoon

Directions:

1. Add oil to a stock pot and heat it over medium heat. Add onion, celery, zucchinis, salt, and zucchini to the oil. Sauté for about 6 to 8 minutes. Stir in thyme and chive and sauté for 1 minute.
2. Add drained tomatoes and cook for 5 to 6 minutes. Pour in broth, water, and quinoa. Stir in red pepper flakes, bay leaves and salt. Bring the mixture to a boil then reduce the heat.
3. Partially cover the lid and let it simmer for 25 minutes. Turn off the pot heat and discard the bay leaves. Add Seville orange juice, salt, and pepper. Serve warm

Nutrition

Calories 336 Fat 14.8g Carbs 40.3g Protein 12.4g Fiber 2.4g

Zucchini and Golden Onion Soup

Preparation Time: 5 minutes | **Cooking Time:** 30 minutes | **Servings:** 4

Ingredients:

o 6-7 zucchinis, chopped into 1/2-inch pieces
o 2-3 golden onion, chopped into 1/2-inch cubes
o 2 shallots, chopped into chunks
o 1 tablespoon olive oil
o 1/4 teaspoons ground turmeric, divided
o 1/4 teaspoons ground cumin, divided

o 1/2 teaspoons dried thyme, divided

o 1/2 teaspoons sea salt

o 2-3 cups vegetable stock

o 2-3 teaspoons lime juice

Directions:

1. Layer 2 baking sheets with tin foil. Preheat oven at 400 degrees. Mix in zucchinis, onion, and shallot to the baking sheets. Top the veggies with spices, salt, and herbs.

2. Drizzle half tablespoon oil and cover the veggies with a foil sheet. Bake for 30 minutes until al dente. Transfer all the ingredients to a blender. Puree the mixture and add the saucepan.

3. Cook for 1 minute. Garnish with cilantro. Serve.

Nutrition

Calories 248 Fat 15.7g Carbs 0.4g Protein 24.9g

Simply Chayote Squash

Preparation Time: 10 minutes | **Cooking Time:** 20 minutes | **Servings:** 1

Ingredients:

o 1 chayote squash

o ¼ teaspoon of coconut oil

o Dash of cayenne pepper

o Dash of sea salt

Directions:

1. Serves as a light snack or part of a dish. Wash and cut chayote squash in half. The seed can by eaten and it has a nice texture.

2. Add chayote, oil, and enough water to cover the chayote in a saucepan. Boil for 20 minutes until fork can penetrate the squash, but the squash should still maintain some firmness.

3. Remove form water. Season it well with cayenne pepper and salt.

Nutrition

Calories 117g Fiber 9.7g Protein 14 g Carbs 3g

Vegetable Medley Sauté

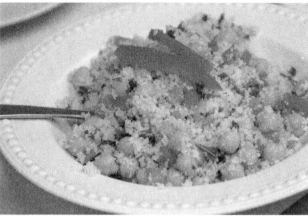

Preparation Time: 10 minutes | **Cooking Time:** 15 minutes | **Servings:** 4

Ingredients:

o 1 cup mushrooms (sliced)

o 1 zucchini (sliced)

o 1 yellow squash (sliced)

o 1 red pepper (chopped)

o 1 green pepper (chopped)

o 2 plum tomatoes (chopped)

o ½ red onion (finely chopped)

o ½ cup chayote (finely chopped)

o 3 tbsp. grape-seed oil or avocado oil

o ⅛ tsp cayenne pepper

o ⅛ tsp sea salt

Directions:

1. Cook the oil in a saucepan over medium heat. Let the oil get hot.

2. Add in mushrooms and onions and sauté for 4 minutes.

3. Add in the rest of the vegetables and spices and sauté for 8-10 minutes.

Nutrition

Calories 115 Fiber 4.9g Protein 21g

Chickpea Butternut Squash

Preparation Time: 10 minutes | **Cooking Time:** 15 minutes | **Servings:** 2

Ingredients:

o 15 oz. cooked chickpeas

o 1 ½ section of a butternut squash

o ¼ plum tomato

o   ¼ cup coconut milk

o   1 cup water (add more water to make thinner soup)

o   Pinch of dill

o   Pinch of all spice

o   Pinch of cayenne pepper

o   ⅛ tsp of sea salt

Directions:

1.   Add all the ingredients to a blender and blend to your desired consistency.

2.   Add the blended ingredients to a saucepan over a medium/high flame until it starts to boil or air bubbles rise.

3.   Adjust it into low heat and cook for 30 minutes.

Nutrition

Calories 110 Fiber 9.7g Protein 11g Carb 11g

Butternut Squash Ginger

Preparation Time: 10 minutes | **Cooking Time:** 15 minutes | **Servings:** 2

Ingredients:

o   1 section of a butternut squash

o   ¼ cup coconut milk

o   1 tbsp. coconut oil

o   3 cups water (add more water to make thinner soup)

o   2 tsp minced fresh ginger

o   1 tbsp. date sugar

o   ½ cup of diced onions

o   1 tsp finely chopped fresh thyme

o   ⅛ tsp of sea salt

o   pinch of all spice

o   pinch of cayenne pepper

Directions:

1.   Peel off the skin and seeds from butternut squash, then chop the squash into medium sized cubes. Add cubes to saucepan and cover cubes with water.

2.   Boil until squash becomes soft. Remove softened squash from water and discard water.

3.   Add butternut squash, coconut milk, and coconut oil to the blender and blend until smooth. Combine the rest of the ingredients and 1 cup of water and blend for a few seconds.

4.   Transfer mix to saucepan and stir in the remaining 2 cups of water to the desired consistency. Add more water if wanted.

5.   Bring to a boil, reduce heat, and let simmer for 15 minutes.

Nutrition

Calories 97 Fiber 6.9g Protein 14g Carbs 8g

Cream of Avocado Mushroom

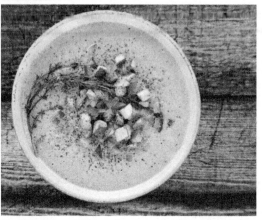

Preparation Time: 5 minutes | **Cooking Time:** 15 minutes | **Servings:** 2-4

Ingredients:

o   2 avocados (scoop out flesh and discard skin)

o   juice of 1 key lime

o   2 cups hot water

o   ⅛ tsp of cayenne pepper

o   ⅛ tsp of sea salt

o   Dash of clove

o   1 tbsp. coconut oil or grape seed oil

o   1 cup of sliced mushrooms

o   1 red bell pepper (diced)

o   ¼ yellow onion (finely chopped)

o   3 plum tomatoes (diced)

o   3 sprigs of fresh thyme leaves

Directions:

1.   Add hot water, avocados, lime juice, cayenne pepper, sea salt, and all spice in a blender. Pulse until smooth.

2.   Heat oil in saucepan over medium and stir in mushrooms, red bell pepper, onion, tomatoes, and thyme until they become soft.

3.   Add in avocado mix to the saucepan and simmer for 5 minutes.

Nutrition

Calories 99 Protein 12g Fibers 5.8g Carbs 14g

Kale, Mushroom, Walnut and Avocado

Preparation Time: 10 minutes | **Cooking Time:** 15 minutes | **Servings:** 2-3

Ingredients:

o   6 kale leaves (chopped)

o   10 crushed walnuts

o   ¼ onion (diced)

o   ¼ red bell pepper (diced)

o   ½ plum tomato (sliced)

o   20 mushrooms slices

o   ½ - 1 tbsp. avocado oil

Dressing:

o   1 tbsp. key lime juice

o   1 tbsp. sesame oil

o   1 plum tomato

o   ⅛ tsp of sea salt

o   ¼ avocado

Directions:

1.   Dressing: Blend the lime juice, sesame oil, plum tomato, salt, and avocado together until smooth. Sauté the mushrooms in the avocado oil.

2.   Let cool afterwards. Mix the kale, walnuts, onion, pepper, tomato, and mushrooms together.

3.   Pour the dressing to the salad then toss it well until it evenly coats the entire salad.

Nutrition

Calories 87 Protein 10g Fiber 4.1 Carbs 15g

Spiced Okra

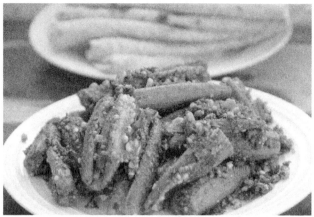

Preparation Time: 10 minutes | **Cooking Time:** 13 minutes | **Servings:** 2

Ingredients:

o   1 tablespoon avocado oil

o   ¾ pound okra pods, 2-inch pieces

o   ½ teaspoon ground cumin

o   ½ teaspoon cayenne powder

o   Sea salt, as required

Directions:

1.   Cook the oil over medium heat and stir fry the okra for about 2 minutes. Reduce the heat to low and cook covered for about 6-8 minutes stirring occasionally.

2.   Add the cumin, cayenne powder and salt and stir to combine. Increase the heat to medium and cook uncovered for about 2-3 minutes more.

3.   Remove from the heat and serve hot.

Nutrition

Calories 81 Total Fat 1.4g Protein 3.5g Carbs 13.5g Fiber 5.9g

Mushroom Curry

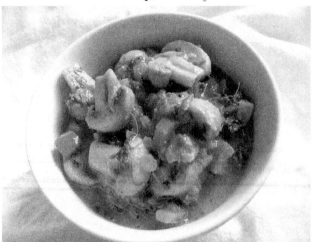

Preparation Time: 15 minutes | **Cooking Time:** 25 minutes | **Servings:** 4

Ingredients:

o   2 cups plum tomatoes, chopped
o   2 tablespoons grapeseed oil
o   1 small onion, chopped finely
o   ¼ teaspoon cayenne powder
o   4 cups fresh button mushrooms, sliced
o   1¼ cups spring water
o   ¼ cup unsweetened coconut milk
o   Sea salt, as required

Directions:

1. In a food processor, add the tomatoes and pulse until a smooth paste form. In a pan, heat the oil over medium heat and sauté the onion for about 5-6 minutes.
2. Add the tomato paste and cook for about 5 minutes. Stir in the mushrooms, water and coconut milk and bring to a boil. Cook for about 10-12 minutes, stirring occasionally.
3. Season it well and remove from the heat. Serve hot.

Nutrition

Calories 126 Total Fat 9.5g Protein 3.7g Carbs 9g Fiber 2.1g

Bell Peppers & Zucchini Stir Fry

Preparation Time: 15 minutes | **Cooking Time:** 15 minutes | **Servings:** 4

Ingredients:

o   2 tablespoons avocado oil
o   1 large onion, cubed

o   4 garlic cloves, minced
o   1 large green bell pepper
o   1 large red bell pepper
o   1 large yellow bell pepper
o   2 cups zucchini, sliced
o   ¼ cup spring water
o   Sea salt, as required
o   Cayenne powder, as required

Directions:

1. Cook the oil over medium heat and sauté the onion and garlic for about 4-5 minutes.
2. Add the vegetables and stir fry for about 4-5 minutes.
3. Add the water and stir fry for about 3-4 minutes more. Serve hot.

Nutrition

Calories 66 Total Fat 1.3g Protein 2.3g Carbs 3.5 Fiber 3g

Yellow Squash & Bell Pepper Bake

Preparation Time: 15 minutes | **Cooking Time:** 20 minutes | **Servings:** 4

Ingredients:

o   2 large yellow squash
o   1 large red bell pepper
o   1 large yellow bell peppers
o   1 onion, cubed
o   1 tablespoon agave nectar
o   2 tablespoons grapeseed oil
o   1 teaspoon cayenne powder
o   Sea salt, as required

Directions:

1. Lightly, grease the baking dish and preheat the oven to 375 degrees.
2. Mix all the ingredients in a bowl.
3. Transfer the vegetable mixture into the prepared baking dish. Bake for about 15-20 minutes. Remove from the oven and serve immediately.

Nutrition

Calories 132 Total Fat 7.6g Protein 2.9g Carbs 16.7g Fiber 3.5g

Mushrooms with Bell Peppers

Preparation Time: 15 minutes | **Cooking Time:** 10 minutes | **Servings:** 4

Ingredients:

o   1 tablespoon grapeseed oil

o   3 cups fresh button mushrooms, sliced

o   ¾ cups red bell peppers

o   ¾ cups green bell peppers strips

o   1½ cup white onions strips

o   2 teaspoons fresh sweet basil

o   2 teaspoons fresh oregano

o   ½ teaspoon cayenne powder

o   Sea salt, as required

o   2 teaspoons onion powder

Directions:

1.   Cook the oil over medium-high heat and sauté the mushrooms, bell peppers and onion for about 5-6 minutes.

2.   Add the herbs and spices and cook for about 2-3 minutes.

3.   Stir in the lime juice and serve hot.

Nutrition

Calories 80 Total Fat 3.9g Protein 2.8g Carbs 10.7g Fiber 2.5g

Bell Peppers & Tomato Casserole

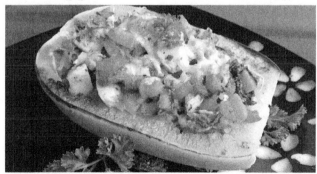

Preparation Time: 15 minutes | **Cooking Time:** 35 minutes | **Serves:** 6

Ingredients:

For Herb Sauce

o   4 garlic cloves, chopped

o   ½ cup fresh parsley, chopped

o   ½ cup fresh cilantro, chopped

o   3 tablespoons avocado oil

o   2 tablespoons fresh key lime juice

o   ½ teaspoon ground cumin

o   ½ teaspoon cayenne powder

o   Sea salt, as required

For Veggies

o   1 large green bell pepper

o   1 large yellow bell pepper

o   1 large orange bell pepper

o   1 large red bell pepper

o   1-pound plum tomatoes wedges

o   2 tablespoons avocado oil

Directions:

1.   Lightly, grease the baking dish and preheat the oven to 350 degrees. For the sauce: transfer all ingredients in food processor and pulse till smooth.

2.   In a large bowl, add the bell peppers and sauce and herb sauce and gently, toss to coat. Transfer the bell pepper mixture into prepared baking dish.

3.   Drizzle with oil. Enclose the baking dish with foil and bake for about 35 minutes. Take off the cover of the baking dish and bake for another 20-30 minutes. Serve hot.

Nutrition

Calories 61 Total Fat 2g Protein 2g Carbs 10.8g Fiber 2.8g

Lentil Kale Soup

Preparation time: 5 minutes | **Cooking time:** 15 minutes | **Servings:** 4

Ingredients:

o   1/2 Onion

o   2 Zucchinis

o   1 rib Celery

o   1 stalk Chive

o   1 cup diced tomatoes

o   1 tsp. dried vegetable broth powder

o   1 tsp. Scazon seasoning

o   1 cup red lentils

o   1 tbsp. Seville orange juice

o   3 cups alkaline water

o   1 bunch kale

Directions:

1. In a greased pan, pour in all the vegetables.
2. Sauté for about 5 minutes, then add the tomatoes, broth, and Scazon seasoning.
3. Mix properly then stir in the red lentils together with water.
4. Cook until the lentils become soft and tender.
5. Add the kale then cook for about 2 minutes.
6. Serve warm with the Seville orange juice.

Nutrition
Calories: 301 Fat: 12.2g Carbs: 15g Protein: 28.8g

Turnip Green Soup

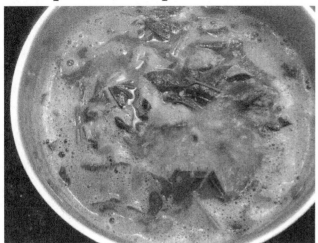

Preparation time: 5 minutes | **Cooking time:** 22 minutes | **Servings:** 2

Ingredients:

o   2 tbsps. Coconut oil

o   1 large, chopped onion

o   3 minced cloves chive

o   2—in piece peeled and minced ginger

o   3 cups bone broth

o   1 medium cubed white turnip

o   1 large, chopped head radish

o   1 bunch chopped kale

o   1 Seville orange, 1/2 zested and juice reserved

o   1/2 tsp. sea salt

o   1 bunch cilantro

Directions:

1. In a skillet, add oil then heat it.
2. Add in the onions as you stir.
3. Sauté for about 7 minutes, then add chive and ginger.
4. Cook for about 1 minute.
5. Add in the turnip, broth, and radish then stir.
6. Bring the soup to boil then reduce the heat to allow it to simmer.
7. Cook for an extra 15 minutes then turn off the heat.
8. Pour in the remaining ingredients.
9. Using a handheld blender, pour the mixture.
10. Garnish with cilantro. Serve warm.

Nutrition

Calories 249 Fat : 11.9g. Crabs : 1.8g. Protein : 35g.

Tangy Lentil Soup

Preparation time: 5 minutes | **Cooking time:** 15 minutes | **Servings:** 4

Ingredients:

o   2 cups picked over and rinsed red lentils

o   1 chopped serrano Chile pepper

o   1 large chopped and roughly tomato

o   1-1/2 inch peeled and grated piece ginger

o   3 finely chopped cloves chive

o   1/4 tsp. ground turmeric

o   Sea salt

o   Topping

o   1/4 cup coconut yogurt

Directions:

1. In a pot add the lentils with enough water to cover the lentils.
2. Boil the lentils then reduce the heat.
3. Cook for about 10 minutes on low heat to simmer.
4. Add the remaining ingredients then stir.
5. Cook until lentils become soft and properly mixed.
6. Garnish a dollop of coconut yogurt.
7. Serve.

Nutrition:

Calories: 248 Fat: 2.4g Carbs: 12.2g Protein: 44.3g

Vegetable Casserole

Preparation time: 5 minutes | **Cooking time:** 1 hr. 30 minutes | **Servings:** 6

Ingredients:

o   2 large peeled and sliced eggplants

o   Sea salt

o   2 large, diced cucumbers

o   2 small diced green peppers

o   1 Small diced red pepper

o   1 Small diced yellow pepper

o   1/4 lb. sliced green beans

o   1/2 cup olive oil

o   2 large chopped sweet onions

o   3 crushed cloves chive

o   2 cubed yellow Squash,

o   20 halved cherry tomatoes

- o 1/2 tsp. sea salt
- o 1/4 tsp. fresh ground pepper
- o 1/4 cup alkaline water
- o 1 cup fresh seasoned breadcrumbs

Directions:

1. Adjust the temperature of your oven to 350°F.
2. Mix the eggplant with salt then keep it aside.
3. Heat a greased skillet then sautés the eggplant until it is evenly browned.
4. Transfer the eggplant to a separate plate.
5. Sauté the onions in the same pan until it becomes soft.
6. Add the chive then stir.
7. Cook for a minute then turn off the heat.
8. Layer a greased casserole dish with the eggplants, yellow squash, cucumbers, peppers, and green beans.
9. Add the onion mixture, tomatoes, pepper, and salt.
10. Sprinkle the seasoned breadcrumbs as toppings.
11. Bake for an hour and 30 minutes.
12. Serve.

Nutrition

Calories: 372 Fat: 11.1g Carbs: 0.9g Protein: 63.5g

Mushroom Leek Soup

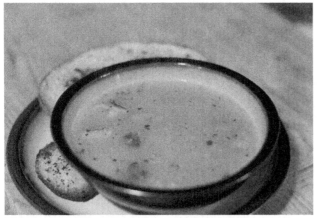

Preparation time: 5 minutes | **Cooking Time:** 8 minutes | **Servings:** 4

Ingredients:

- o 3 tbsps. Divided vegetable oil
- o 2—3/4 cups finely chopped leeks
- o 3 finely minced chive stalks
- o 7 cups cleaned and sliced assorted mushrooms
- o 5 tbsps. Coconut flour

- o 3/4 tsp. sea salt
- o 1/2 tsp. ground black pepper
- o 1 tbsp. finely minced fresh dill
- o 3 cups vegetable broth
- o 2/3 cup coconut cream
- o 1/2 cup coconut milk
- o 1—1/2 tbsps. Sherry vinegar

Directions:

1. Preheat oil in a Dutch oven, then sauté the leeks and chive until they become soft.
2. Add in the mushrooms then stir.
3. Sauté for about 10 minutes.
4. Add pepper, dill, flour, and salt.
5. Mix properly then cook for about 2 minutes.
6. Pour in the broth then cook to boil.
7. Reduce the heat in the oven then add the remaining ingredients.
8. Serve warm with coconut flour bread.

Nutrition

Calories: 127 Fat: 3.5g Carbs: 3.6g Protein: 21.5g

Red Lentil Squash Soup

Preparation time: 5 minutes | **Cooking time:** 4 minutes | **Servings:** 4

Ingredients:

- o 1 chopped yellow onion
- o 2 tbsps. Olive oil
- o 1 large, diced butternut squash
- o 1—1/2 cups red lentils
- o 2 tsps. Dried sage
- o 7 cups vegetable broth
- o Mineral sea salt & white or fresh cracked pepper

Directions:

1. Preheat the oil in a stockpot.
2. Add the onions then cook for about 5 minutes.
3. Add in the sage and squash.
4. Cook for 5 minutes.
5. Add broth, pepper, lentils, and salt.
6. Cook gradually for 30 minutes on low heat.
7. Pour the mixture using a handheld blender.
8. Garnish with cilantro.
9. Serve.

Nutrition

Calories: 323   Fat: 7.5g Carbs: 21.4g   Protein: 10.1g

Calories: 332 Fat: 7.5g Carbs: 19.4g Protein: 3.1g

Cauliflower Potato Curry

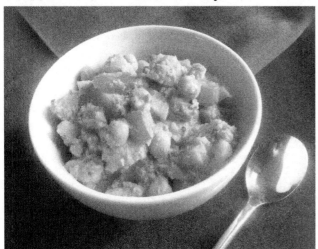

Preparation time: 10 minutes | **Cooking time:** 35 minutes | **Servings:** 4

Ingredients:

o   2 tbsps. Vegetable oil

o   1 large, chopped onion

o   A large, grated piece of ginger

o   3 finely chopped chive stalks

o   1/2 tsp. turmeric

o   1 tsp. ground cumin

o   1 tsp. curry powder

o   1 cup chopped tomatoes

o   1/2 tsp. sugar

o   1 florets cauliflower

o   2 chopped potatoes

o   1 small halved lengthways green chili

o   A squeeze Seville orange juice

o   Handful roughly chopped coriander

Directions:

1.   Add the onion to a greased skillet then sauté until soft.

2.   Add all the spices in the skillet then stir.

3.   Add the cauliflower and potatoes.

4.   Sauté for about 5 minutes, then add green chilies tomatoes, and sugar.

5.   Cover then cook for about 30 minutes.

6.   Serve warm with the coriander and Seville orange juice.

Nutrition

Vegetable Bean Curry

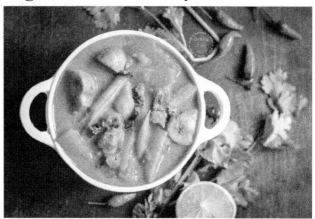

Preparation time: 5 minutes | **Cooking time:** 6 hours.

Servings: 8

Ingredients:

o   1 finely chopped onion

o   4 chopped chive stalks

o   3 tsps. Coriander powder

o   1/2 tsp. cinnamon powder

o   1 tsp. ginger powder

o   1 tsp. turmeric powder

o   1/2 tsp. cayenne pepper

o   2 tbsps. Tomato paste

o   1 tbsp. avocado oil

o   2 cans, 15 ounces each, well rinsed and drained lima beans

o   3 cups cubed and peeled turnips

o   3 cups fresh cauliflower florets

o   4 medium diced zucchinis

o   2 medium seeded and chopped tomatoes

o   2 cups vegetable broth

o   1 cup light coconut milk

o   1/2 tsp. pepper

o   1/4 tsp. sea salt

Directions:

1.   In a slow cooker, preheat the oil then add all the vegetables.

2.   Add in the remaining ingredients then stir.

3.   Cook for about 6 hours on low temperature.

4.   Serve warm.

Nutrition

Calories: 403 Fat: 12.5g   Carbs: 21.4g Protein: 8.1g

Wild Mushroom Soup

Preparation time: 10 minutes | **Cooking time:** 15 minutes | **Servings:** 4

Ingredients:

o   4 oz. walnut butter

o   1 chopped shallot

o   5 oz. chopped portabella mushrooms

o   5 oz. chopped oyster mushrooms

o   5 oz. chopped shiitake mushrooms

o   1 minced chive clove

o   1/2 tsp. dried thyme

o   3 cups alkaline water

o   1 vegetable bouillon cube

o   1 cup coconut cream

o   1/2 lb. chopped celery root

o   1 tbsp. white wine vinegar

o   Fresh cilantro

Directions:

1.   In a cooking pan, melt the butter over medium heat.

2.   Add the vegetables into the pan then sauté until golden brown.

3.   Add the remaining ingredients to the pan then properly mix it.

4.   Boil the mixture.

5.   Simmer it for 15 minutes on low heat.

6.   Add the cream to the soup then pour it using a hand-held blender.

7.   Serve warm with the chopped cilantro as toppings.

Nutrition

Calories: 243 Fat: 7.5g Carbs: 14.4g Protein: 10.1g

Bok Choy Soup

Preparation time: 5 minutes | **Cooking time:** 10 minutes | **Servings:** 2

Ingredients:

o   1 cup chopped Bok Choy

o   3 cups vegetable broth

o   2 peeled and sliced zucchinis

o   1/2 cup cooked hemp seed

o   1 roughly chopped bunch radish

Directions:

1.   In a pan, mix the ingredients over moderate heat.

2.   Let it simmer then cook it for about 10 minutes until the vegetables become tender.

3.   Serve.

Nutrition:

Calories: 172 kcal Fat: 3.5g Carbs: 38.5g Protein: 11.7g

Grilled Vegetable Stack

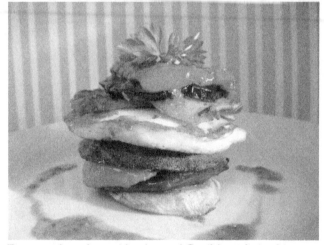

Preparation time: 10 minutes | **Cooking time:** 20 minutes | **Servings:** 2

Ingredients:

o   1/2 zucchini, sliced into slices about 1/4—inch thick

o   2 stemmed Portobello mushrooms with the gills removed

o   1 tsp. divided sea salt

o   1/2 cup divided hummus

o   1 peeled and sliced red onion

o   1 seeded red bell pepper, sliced lengthwise

o   1 seeded yellow bell pepper, sliced lengthwise

Directions:

1.   Adjust the temperature of your broiler or grill.

2.   Grill the mushroom caps over coal or gas flame.

3.   Add the yellow and red bell peppers, onion, and zucchini for about 20 minutes as you turn it occasionally.

4.   Fill the mushroom cap with 1/4 cup of hummus.

5.   Top it with some onion, yellow peppers, red and zucchini.

6.   Add salt to season then set it aside.

7. Redo the process with the second mushroom cap and the remaining ingredients. Serve

Nutrition

Calories: 179 Fat: 3.1g Carbs: 15.7g Protein: 3.9g

Date Night Chive Bake

Preparation time: 10 minutes | **Cooking time:** 30 minutes | **Servings:** 2

Ingredients:

o 4 peeled and sliced lengthwise zucchinis

o 1 lb. Radish chopped into bite-size pieces

o 2 tsps. Seville orange zest

o 3 peeled and chopped chive heads cloves

o 2 tbsps. Coconut oil

o 1 cup vegetable broth

o 1/4 tsps. Mustard powder

o 1 tsp. sea salt

Directions:

1. Adjust the temperature of the oven to 400°F.
2. In a separate bowl, mix all the ingredients.
3. Spread the mixture in a baking pan evenly.
4. Cover the mixture with a piece of aluminum foil then place it in the oven.
5. Bake the mixture for about 30 minutes as you stir it once halfway through the cooking time.
6. Serve.

Nutrition

Calories: 270 Fat: 15.2g Carbs: 28.1g Protein: 11.6g

Champions Chili

Preparation time: 5 minutes | **Cooking time:** 25 minutes | **Servings:** 4

Ingredients:

o 1 cup diced red bell pepper

o 1 chopped onion

o 2 finely chopped chive stalks

o 2 cups sprouted pinto beans

o 1/4 cup fresh organic cilantro

o 1/4 cup organic salsa

o 8 oz. jar organic pasta sauce

o 2 tbsps. Barbecue sauce

o Dash of ground cumin

o Dash of chili powder

Directions:

1. Apply some non-stick cooking spray to a pot.
2. Place the pot over a moderate heat then sauté the onion for about 5 minutes.
3. Add in the ingredients then stir.
4. Simmer for about 20 minutes.
5. Serve.

Nutrition

Calories: 101 Fat: 2.7g Carbs: 18.5g Protein: 3.9g

Dinner Recipes

Easy Cilantro Lime Quinoa

Preparation Time: 5 minutes | **Cooking Time:** 15 minutes | **Servings:** 6

Ingredients:

o   1 cup quinoa, rinsed and drained

o   1/2 cup fresh cilantro, chopped

o   1 lime zest, grated

o   2 tbsp. fresh lime juice

o   1 1/4 cups filtered alkaline water

o   Sea salt

Directions:

1. Add quinoa & water to the instant pot and stir well.
2. Seal pot with the lid and select manual mode and set timer for 5 minutes.
3. When finished, allow releasing pressure naturally, then open the lid.
4. Stir in cilantro, lime zest, and lime juice.
5. Season with salt and serve.

Nutrition

Calories: 105 Fat: 1.7 g Carbs: 18.3 g Protein: 4 g

Spinach Quinoa

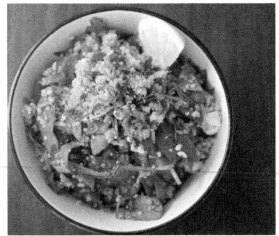

Preparation Time: 10 minutes | **Cooking Time:** 25 minutes | **Servings:** 4

Ingredients:

o   1 cup quinoa

o   2 cups fresh spinach, chopped

o   1 1/2 cups filtered alkaline water

o   1 sweet potato, peeled and cubed

o   1 tsp coriander powder

o   1 top turmeric

o   1 tsp cumin seeds

o   1 tsp fresh ginger, grated

o   2 garlic cloves, chopped

o   1 cup onion, chopped

o   2 tbsp. olive oil

o   1 fresh lime juice

o   Pepper

o   Salt

Directions:

1. Add oil to the instant pot and set the pot on sauté mode.
2. Add the onion in olive oil and sauté for 2 minutes or until the onion is softened.
3. Add garlic, ginger, spices, and quinoa, and cook for 3-4 minutes.
4. Add spinach, sweet potatoes, and water and stir well.
5. Seal pot w/ lid and cook on manual high pressure for 2 minutes.
6. When finished, allow releasing pressure naturally, then open the lid.
7. Add lime juice and stir well.
8. Serve and enjoy.

Nutrition

Calories: 268 Fat: 9.9 g Carbohydrates: 38.8 g Sugar: 3.4 g Protein: 7.6 g Cholesterol: 0 mg

Healthy Broccoli Asparagus Soup

Preparation Time: 15 minutes | **Cooking Time:** 28 minutes | **Servings:** 6

Ingredients:

o   2 cups broccoli florets, chopped

o   15 asparagus spears, ends trimmed and chopped

o   1 tsp dried oregano

o   1 tbsp. fresh thyme leaves

o   1/2 cup unsweetened almond milk

o   3 1/2 cups filtered alkaline water

o   2 cups cauliflower florets, chopped

o   2 tsp garlic, chopped

o   1 cup onion, chopped

o   2 tbsp. olive oil

o   Pepper

o   Salt

Directions:

1. Add oil to the instant pot and set the pot on sauté mode.

2. Add onion to the olive oil and sauté until onion is softened.

3. Add garlic and sauté for 30 seconds.

4. Add all vegetables and water and stir well.

5. Seal pot with lid and cook on manual mode for 3 minutes.

6. When finished, allow releasing pressure naturally, then open the lid.

7. Puree the soup using an immersion blender.

8. Stir in almond milk, herbs, pepper, and salt.

9. Serve and enjoy.

Nutrition

Calories: 85 Fat: 5.2 g Carbohydrates: 8.8 g Sugar: 3.3 g Protein: 3.3 g Cholesterol: 0 mg

Creamy Asparagus Soup

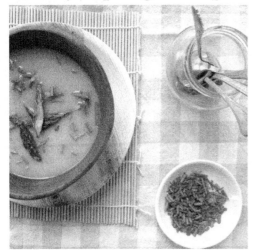

Preparation Time: 10 minutes | **Cooking Time:** 40 minutes | **Servings:** 6

Ingredients:

o   2 lbs. fresh asparagus, cut off woody stems

o   1/4 tsp lime zest

o   2 tbsp. lime juice

o   14 oz. coconut milk

o   1 tsp dried thyme

o   1/2 tsp oregano

o   1/2 tsp sage

o   1 1/2 cups filtered alkaline water

o   1 cauliflower head, cut into florets

o   1 tbsp. garlic, minced

o   1 leek, sliced

o   3 tbsp. coconut oil

o   Pinch of Himalayan salt

Directions:

1. Preheat oven to 400 F/ 200 C.

2. Line baking tray w/ parchment paper and set aside.

3. Arrange asparagus spears on a baking tray. Drizzle w/ 2 tablespoons of coconut oil and sprinkle with salt, thyme, oregano, and sage.

4. Bake in preheated oven for 20-25 minutes.

5. Add remaining oil to the instant pot and set the pot on sauté mode.

6. Add garlic and leek to the pot and sauté for 2-3 minutes.

7. Add cauliflower florets and water to the pot and stir well.

8. Seal pot with a lid and select steam mode and set timer for 4 minutes.

9. When finished, release pressure using the quick-release method.

10. Add roasted asparagus, lime zest, lime juice, and coconut milk and stir well.

11. Puree the soup using an immersion blender.

12. Serve and enjoy.

Nutrition:

Calories: 265 Fat: 22.9 g Carbohydrates: 14.7 g Sugar: 6.7 g Protein: 6.1 g Cholesterol: 0 mg

Spicy Eggplant

Preparation Time: 15 minutes | **Cooking Time:** 5 minutes | **Servings:** 4

Ingredients:

o   1 eggplant, cut into 1-inch cubes

o   1/2 cup filtered alkaline water

o   1 cup tomato, chopped

o   1/2 tsp Italian seasoning

o   1 tsp paprika

o   1/2 tsp red pepper

o   1 tsp garlic powder

o   2 tbsp. extra virgin olive oil

o   1/4 tsp sea salt

Directions:

1. Add eggplant and water into the instant pot.

2. Seal pot with lid and cook on manual high pressure for 5 minutes.

3. When finished, release pressure using the quick-release method, then open the lid. Drain eggplant well.

4. Add oil to the instant pot and set the pot on sauté mode.

5. Return eggplant in the pot along with tomato, Italian seasoning, paprika, red pepper, garlic powder, and salt and stir until combined.

6. Cook on sauté mode for 5 minutes. Stir occasionally.

7. Serve and enjoy.

Nutrition

Calories: 107 Fat: 7.6 g Carbohydrates: 10.5 g Sugar: 5.6 g Protein: 1.9 g Cholesterol: 0 mg

Brussels Sprouts & Carrots

Preparation Time: 10 minutes | **Cooking Time:** 5 minutes | **Servings:** 6

Ingredients:

o   1 1/2 lb. Brussels sprouts, trimmed and cut in half

o   4 carrots, peel and cut into thick slices

o   1 tsp olive oil

o   1/2 cup filtered alkaline water

o   1 tbsp. dried parsley

o   1/4 tsp garlic, chopped

o   1/4 tsp pepper

o   1/4 tsp sea salt

Directions:

1. Add all ingredients into an instant pot and stir well.

2. Seal pot with lid and cook on manual high pressure for 2 minutes.

3. When finished, release pressure using the quick-release method than open the lid.

4. Stir well and serve.

Nutrition

Calories: 73 Fat: 1.2 g Carbohydrates: 14.5 g Sugar: 4.5 g Protein: 4.2 g Cholesterol: 0 mg

Cajun Seasoned Zucchini

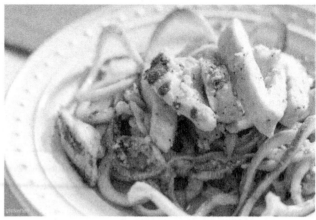

Preparation Time: 8 minutes | **Cooking Time:** 2 minutes | **Servings:** 2

Ingredients:

o   4 zucchinis, sliced

o   1 tsp garlic powder

o   1 tsp paprika

o   2 tbsp. Cajun seasoning

o   1/2 cup filtered alkaline water

o   1 tbsp. olive oil

Directions:

1. Add all ingredients into an instant pot and stir well.

2. Seal pot with lid and cook on low pressure for 1 minute.

3. When finished, release pressure using the quick-release method than open the lid.

4. Stir well and serve.

Nutrition

Calories: 130 Fat: 7.9 g Carbohydrates: 14.7 g Sugar: 7.2 g Protein: 5.3 g Cholesterol: 0 mg

Fried Cabbage

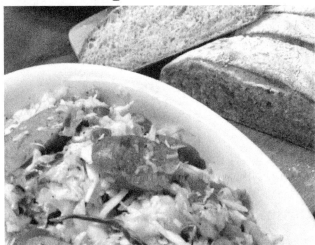

Preparation Time: 10 minutes | **Cooking Time:** 3 minutes | **Serve:** 6

Ingredients:

o   1 head cabbage, chopped

o   1/2 tsp chili powder

o   1/2 onion, diced

o   1/2 tsp paprika

o   1 onion, chopped

o   1 cup filtered alkaline water

o   2 tbsp. olive oil

o   1/2 tsp sea salt

Directions:

1.   Add olive oil into the instant pot and set the pot on sauté mode.

2.   Add the onion in olive oil and sauté until softened.

3.   Add remaining ingredients and stir to combine.

4.   Seal pot with lid and cook on high pressure for 3 minutes.

5.   When finished, release pressure using the quick-release method than open the lid.

6.   Stir well and serve.

Nutrition

Calories: 75 Fat: 4.9 g Carbohydrates: 8 g Sugar: 4.2 g Protein: 1.7 g Cholesterol: 0 mg

Tofu Curry

Preparation Time: 10 minutes | **Cooking Time:** 4 hours | **Servings:** 4

Ingredients:

o   1 cup firm tofu, diced

o   2 tsp garlic cloves, minced

o   1 onion, chopped

o   8 oz. tomato puree

o   2 cups bell pepper, chopped

o   1 tbsp. garam masala

o   2 tbsp. olive oil

o   1 tbsp. curry powder

o   10 oz. coconut milk

o   1 1/2 tsp sea salt

Directions:

1.   Add all ingredients except tofu in a blender and blend until smooth.

2.   Pour blended mixture into the instant pot.

3.   Add tofu to a pot and stir well to coat.

4.   Seal the pot with a lid and select slow cook mode and set the timer for 4 hours.

5.   Stir well and serve.

Nutrition

Calories: 326 Fat: 27.1 g Carbohydrates: 18.5 g Sugar: 9.7 g Protein: 8.9 g Cholesterol: 0 mg

Whole Cauliflower with Gravy

Preparation Time: 10 minutes | **Cooking Time:** 15 minutes | **Servings:** 5

Ingredients:

o   1 large cauliflower head, cut bottom leaves

For marinade:

o   1 tsp paprika 1/2 tbsp. olive oil

o   tbsp. fresh parsley, chopped

o   1 tbsp. fresh thyme

o   3 garlic cloves

o   Pepper

o   Salt

For gravy:

o   1/2 tbsp. lime juice

o   1/2 tsp thyme

o   1 1/2 cups filtered alkaline water

o   2 garlic cloves

o   1 tsp olive oil

o   1 onion, diced

Directions:

1.   In a small bowl, mix all marinade ingredients.

2.   Rub marinade evenly all over cauliflower head.

3. For the gravy: add oil in an instant pot and set the pot on sauté mode.

4. Add garlic and onion in olive oil and sauté until onion is softened.

5. Add water, lemon juice, and thyme and stir well.

6. Place trivet in the instant pot. Place cauliflower head on a trivet.

7. Seal pot with lid and cook on manual high pressure for 3 minutes.

8. When finished, allow releasing pressure naturally for 5 minutes, then release using a quick-release method.

9. Transfer cauliflower head to an oven-safe dish and broil for 3-4 minutes.

10. Puree the instant pot gravy using an immersion hand blender until smooth.

11. Set instant pot on sauté mode and cook the gravy for 3-4 minutes.

12. Serve cauliflower with gravy.

Nutrition

Calories: 79 Fat: 2.7 g Carbohydrates: 12.7 g Sugar: 5.1 g Protein: 3.9 g Cholesterol: 0 mg

Alkaline Carrot Soup with Fresh Mushrooms

Preparation Time: 10 minutes | **Cooking Time:** 20 minutes | **Servings:** 1-2

Ingredients:

o 4 mid-sized carrots

o 4 mid-sized potatoes

o 10 enormous new mushrooms (champignons or chanterelles)

o 1/2 white onion

o 2 tbsp. olive oil (cold squeezed, additional virgin)

o 3 cups vegetable stock

o 2 tbsp. parsley, new and cleaved

o Salt and new white pepper

Directions:

1. Wash and strip carrots and potatoes and dice them.

2. Warmth up vegetable stock in a pot on medium warmth and cook carrots and potatoes for around 15 minutes.

3. Meanwhile, finely shape onion and braise them in a container with olive oil for around 3 minutes.

4. Wash mushrooms, slice them to wanted size, and add to the container, cooking approx., an additional 5 minutes, blending at times.

5. Utilizing a submersion blender, Blend carrots, vegetable stock, and potatoes, and putting the skillet's substance into a pot.

6. When nearly done, season with parsley, salt, and pepper and serve hot.

7. Appreciate this alkalizing soup!

Nutrition

Calories: 75 Carb: 13g Fat: 1.8g Protein: 1 g

Pumpkin and White Bean Soup with Sage

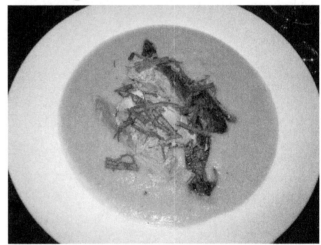

Preparation Time: 10 minutes | **Cooking Time:** 40 minutes | **Servings:** 3-4

Ingredients:

o 1 1/2-pound pumpkin

o 1/2-pound yams

o 1/2-pound white beans

o 1 onion

o 2 cloves of garlic

o 1 tbsp. of cold squeezed additional virgin olive oil

o 1 tbsp. of spices (your top picks)

o 1 tbsp. of sage

o 1 1/2-quart water (best: antacid water)

o A spot of ocean salt and pepper

Directions:

1. Cut the pumpkin and potatoes in shapes, cut the onion, and cut the garlic, the spices, and the sage in fine pieces.

2. Sautéed food, the onion, and garlic in some olive oil for two or three minutes.

3. Include the potatoes, pumpkin, spices, and sage and fry for an additional 5 minutes.

4. At that point, include the water and cook for around 30 minutes (spread the pot with a top) until vegetables are delicate.

5. At long last, include the beans and some salt and pepper. Cook for an additional 5 minutes and serve right away.

6. Prepared!! Appreciate this antacid soup. Alkalizing tasty!

Nutrition:

Calories: 78 Carbohydrates: 12g Fat 3g Proteins 18g

Alkaline Carrot Soup with Millet

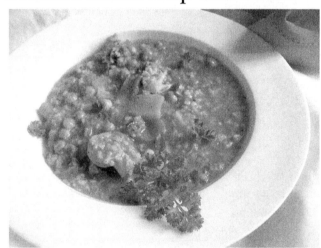

Preparation Time: 7 minutes | **Cooking Time:** 40 minutes | **Servings:** 3-4

Ingredients:

o 2 cups cauliflower pieces

o 1 cup potatoes, cubed

o 2 cups vegetable stock (without yeast)

o 3 tbsp. Swiss Emmenthal cheddar, cubed

o 2 tbsp. new chives

o 1 tbsp. pumpkin seeds

o 1 touch of nutmeg and cayenne pepper

Directions:

1. Cook cauliflower and potato in vegetable stock until delicate and Blend with a blender.

2. Season the soup with nutmeg and cayenne, and possibly somewhat salt and pepper.

3. Include Emmenthal cheddar and chives and mix a couple of moments until the soup is smooth and prepared to serve.

4. Enhancement with pumpkin seeds.

Nutrition

Calories: 65 Carbohydrates: 15g Fat: 1g Protein: 2g

Alkaline Pumpkin Coconut Soup

Preparation Time: 10 minutes | **Cooking Time:** 15 minutes | **Servings:** 3-4

Ingredients:

o 2lb pumpkin

o 6 cups water (best: soluble water delivered with a water ionizer) 1 cup low-Fat: coconut milk

o 5 ounces potatoes

o 2 major onions

o 3 ounces leek

o 1 bunch of new parsley

o 1 touch of nutmeg

o 1 touch of cayenne pepper

o 1 tsp. ocean salt or natural salt

o 4 tbsp. cold squeezed additional virgin olive oil

Directions:

1. As a matter of first importance: cut the onions, the pumpkin, the potatoes just as the hole into little pieces.

2. At that point, heat the olive oil in a major pot and sauté the onions for a couple of moments.

3. At that point, include the water and heat up the pumpkin, potatoes, and the leek until delicate.

4. Include coconut milk.

5. Presently utilize a hand blender and puree for around 1 moment. The soup should turn out to be extremely velvety.

6. Season with salt, pepper, and nutmeg. Lastly, include the parsley. 7. Appreciate this alkalizing pumpkin soup, hot or cold!

Nutrition

Calories: 88 Carbohydrates: 23g Fat: 2.5 g Protein: 1.8g

Cold Cauliflower-Coconut Soup

Preparation Time: 7 minutes | **Cooking Time:** 20 minutes | **Servings:** 3-4

Ingredients:

o 1 pound (450g) new cauliflower

o   1 1/4 cup (300ml) unsweetened coconut milk

o   1 cup water (best: antacid water)

o   2 tbsp. new lime juice

o   1/3 cup cold squeezed additional virgin olive oil

o   1 cup new coriander leaves, slashed

o   Spot of salt and cayenne pepper

o   1 bunch of unsweetened coconut chips

Directions:

1.   Steam cauliflower for around 10 minutes.

2.   At that point, set up the cauliflower with coconut milk and water in a food processor and procedure until extremely smooth.

3.   Include new lime squeeze, salt and pepper, a large portion of the cleaved coriander, and the oil and blend for an additional couple of moments.

4.   Pour in soup bowls and embellishment with coriander and coconut chips. Appreciate!

Nutrition

Calories: 65 Carb: 11g Fat: 0.3g Protein: 1.5g

Jicama & Sweet Pepper

Preparation time: 10 minutes | **Cooking time:** 45 minutes | **Servings:** 4

Ingredients:

o   6 carrots, peeled & shredded

o   1 small jicama, peeled & shredded

o   12 mini sweet peppers thinly sliced, or reg. sweet peppers

o   1 cup cilantro, chopped or snipped

o   1/4 cup extra virgin olive oil

o   2 tablespoons agave syrup

o   1 large clove garlic, crushed

o   1/2 teaspoon cumin

o   1/4 teaspoon cayenne or to taste

o   1/8 teaspoon sea salt

Directions:

1.   Mix olive oil with agave, spices, and garlic in a bowl.

2.   Toss in the chopped vegetables and garnish with cilantro.

3.   Serve.

Nutrition

Calories: 338 Fat: 3.8g Carb: 39.8g Protein: 14.8g

Beans and Broccoli in Sauce

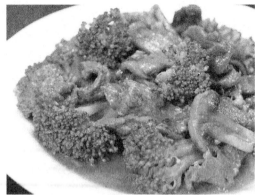

Preparation time: 10 minutes | **Cooking time:** 10 minutes | **Servings:** 4

Ingredients:

o   ¼ cup avocado oil

o   12 white mushrooms, finely chopped

o   1 yellow onion, finely chopped

o   8 garlic cloves, minced

o   A pinch of sea salt

o   2 (14-ounce) cans coconut milk

o   1 cup low-sodium vegetable stock

o   8 cups coarsely chopped broccoli

o   1 cup canned navy beans, drained and rinsed

o   Freshly ground black pepper, for seasoning

Directions:

1.   Heat the oil in a pot.

2.   Add the onion, mushrooms, garlic, and salt. Sauté for 5 minutes.

3.   Stir in the coconut milk and stock and bring to a boil.

4.   Add the broccoli and beans.

5.   Cover the pot and lower heat. Simmer for 5 minutes.

6.   Season with pepper and serve.

Nutrition

Calories: 531 Fat: 33g Carb: 48g Protein: 19g

Sesame Mixed Noodles

Preparation time: 10 minutes | **Cooking time:** 0 minutes | **Servings:** 4

Ingredients:

o   1/2 daikon radish, julienned

o   2 small yellow zucchinis, julienned or spiral noodle cut

o   2 carrots, julienned, about

o   1 cup Snow peas, thinly slivered, about 1 cup

- o   2 cups arugula
- o   1/2 bunch cilantro, chopped

For the sauce

- o   3/4 cup tahini, preferably raw but either will do
- o   1/4 cup Bragg's liquid aminos
- o   1 teaspoon ginger, freshly grated
- o   1/2 teaspoon toasted sesame oil, optional
- o   1-2 tablespoon water
- o   For garnish:
- o   1 mango, thinly slivered
- o   black sesame seeds

Directions:

1. Mix all the herbs and vegetables in a bowl.
2. Combine all the remaining ingredients and add water in the end gradually while mixing well.
3. Garnish with sesame seeds and cilantro.
4. Serve.

Nutrition

Calories: 338 Fat: 3.7g Carb: 8.2g Protein: 5.4g

Citrus Quinoa with Avocado

Preparation time: 10 minutes | **Cooking time:** 20 minutes | **Servings:** 4

Ingredients:

- o   1 cup quinoa
- o   2 cups low-sodium vegetable stock
- o   Juice of 2 limes
- o   2 tbsp. extra-virgin olive oil
- o   2 tsp. apple cider vinegar
- o   1 shallot, finely chopped
- o   4 garlic cloves, minced
- o   2 avocados, pitted, halved, and mashed
- o   A pinch of sea salt
- o   Red pepper flakes, for garnish

Directions:

1. In a pot, combine the quinoa and stock.
2. Cover the pot and bring to a boil over high heat. Lower the heat and cook for 20 minutes or until the quinoa is cooked.
3. Then stir in the oil, lime juice, vinegar, shallot, garlic, avocados, and salt. Mix well.
4. Garnish with a sprinkle of red pepper flakes and serve.

Nutrition

Calories: 424 Fat: 16g Carb: 50g Protein: 11g

Three Bean Chili

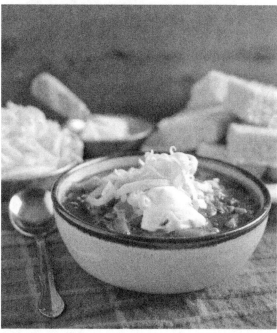

Preparation time: 10 minutes | **Cooking time:** 25 minutes | **Servings:** 4

Ingredients:

- o   1 (28-ounce) can diced tomatoes
- o   ¼ yellow onion, finely chopped
- o   2 garlic cloves, minced
- o   1½ tbsp. chili powder
- o   1 tbsp. cacao powder
- o   1 tsp. pure maple syrup
- o   Pinch sea salt
- o   1 (14-ounce) can kidney beans, drained and rinsed
- o   ½ (14-ounce) can black beans, drained and rinsed
- o   ½ (14-ounce) can navy beans, drained and rinsed

Directions:

1. In a pot, combine the onion, tomatoes, garlic, chili powder, cacao powder, maple syrup, and salt.
2. Place the pot over medium heat and bring to a boil.
3. Add the kidney beans, black beans, and navy beans.
4. Cover the pot. Reduce the heat and simmer for 20 minutes.
5. Serve.

Nutrition

Calories: 264 Fat: 7g Carb: 61g Protein: 13g

Vegetable Stew

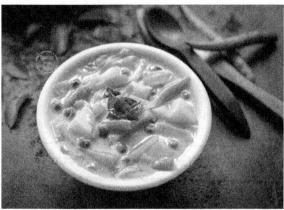

Preparation time: 10 minutes | **Cooking time:** 30 minutes | **Servings:** 4

Ingredients:

o 3 cups low-sodium vegetable stock

o 2 (28-ounce) cans diced tomatoes

o 1 (14-ounce) can black beans, drained and rinsed

o 1 yellow onion, finely chopped

o 1 yam, coarsely chopped

o 2 tsp. ground cumin

o 2 tsp. curry powder

o 1 tsp. ground cinnamon

o ½ tsp. ground ginger

o A pinch of sea salt, plus more for seasoning

Directions:

1. In a pot, combine the stock, tomatoes, beans, onion, yam, cumin, curry powder, cinnamon, ginger, and salt.
2. Cover the pot and bring to a boil over high heat.
3. Lower the heat and simmer for 25 minutes.
4. Adjust seasoning and serve.

Nutrition

Calories: 507 Fat: 23g Carb: 117g Protein: 26g

Asparagus Risotto

Preparation time: 15 minutes | **Cooking time:** 45 minutes | **Servings:** 4

Ingredients:

o 15-20 fresh asparagus spears, trimmed and cut into 1½-inch pieces

o 2 tbsp olive oil

o 1 cup yellow onion, chopped

o 1 garlic clove, minced

o 1 cup Arborio rice

o 1 tbsp fresh lemon zest, grated finely

o 2 tbsp fresh lemon juice

o 5½ cups hot vegetable broth

o 1 tbsp fresh parsley, chopped

o ¼ cup nutritional yeast

o Sea salt and freshly ground black pepper, to taste

Directions:

1. Boil water in a medium pan then add asparagus and cook for about 3 minutes.
2. Drain the asparagus and rinse under cold running water.
3. Drain well and set aside.
4. In a large pan, heat oil over medium heat and sauté the onion for about 5 minutes.
5. Add the garlic and sauté for about 1 minute.
6. Add the rice and stir fry for about 2 minutes.
7. Add the lemon zest, lemon juice, and ½ cup of broth and cook for about 3 minutes or until all the liquid is absorbed, stirring gently.
8. Add 1 cup of broth and cook until all the broth is absorbed, stirring occasionally.
9. Repeat this process by adding ¾ cup of broth at a time until all the broth is absorbed, stirring occasionally. (This procedure will take about 20-30 minutes.)
10. Stir in the cooked asparagus and remaining ingredients and cook for about 4 minutes.
11. Serve hot.

Nutrition

Calories: 353 Fat: 9.6g Carb: 49.2g Protein: 16.8g

Quinoa with Spring Vegetables

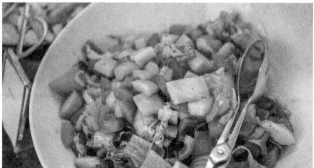

Preparation time: 10 minutes | **Cooking time:** 30 minutes | **Servings:** 4

Ingredients:

o 1 (28-ounce) can crushed tomatoes

o   1 cup low-sodium vegetable stock

o   1 cup quinoa

o   1 tbsp. dried basil

o   A pinch of sea salt, plus more for seasoning

o   1 cup halved snap peas

o   ½ cup coarsely chopped yellow bell peppers

o   ½ cup thinly sliced white mushrooms

o   Freshly ground black pepper, for seasoning

Directions:

1. In a pot, combine the stock, tomatoes, quinoa, basil, and salt.
2. Cover and bring to a boil over high heat.
3. Reduce the heat to low. Cook on low heat for 20 minutes.
4. Stir in the peas, peppers, and mushrooms.
5. Cover and let simmer for 5 to 10 minutes or until cooked.
6. Adjust seasoning and serve.

Nutrition

Calories: 249 Fat: 2g Carb: 49g Protein: 11g

Spicy Vegetable Chili

Preparation time: 10 minutes | **Cooking time:** 25 minutes | **Servings:** 4

Ingredients:

o   1 yam, peeled and cut into ½-inch chunks

o   1 zucchini, coarsely chopped

o   1 white onion, coarsely chopped

o   1 cup thinly sliced white mushrooms

o   1 (28-ounce) can diced tomatoes

o   1 tbsp. chili powder

o   1 tsp. dried oregano

o   1 tsp. ground cumin

o   ½ tsp. paprika

o   A pinch of sea salt, plus more for seasoning

Directions:

1. In a pot, combine the zucchini, yam, onion, mushrooms, tomatoes, chili powder, oregano, cumin, paprika, and salt.
2. Cover and bring to a boil over high heat.
3. Lower the heat and simmer for 25 minutes.
4. Adjust seasoning and serve.

Nutrition

Calories: 219 Fat: 0g Carb: 56g Protein: 3 g

Sweet Potato and Quinoa Stew

Preparation time: 10 minutes

Cooking time: 25 minutes

Servings: 4

Ingredients:

o   1 cup quinoa

o   2 cups low-sodium vegetable stock

o   2 (28-ounce) cans diced tomatoes

o   1 sweet potato, peeled and cut into ½-inch chunks

o   1 white onion, chopped

o   4 white mushrooms, thinly sliced

o   4 garlic cloves, minced

o   2½ tbsp. ground cumin

o   2½ tsp. coriander

o   A pinch of sea salt

Directions:

1. In a pot, combine the quinoa, stock, tomatoes, sweet potato, onion, mushrooms, garlic, cumin, coriander, and salt.
2. Cover the pot and bring to a boil.
3. Lower the heat to low and simmer for 25 minutes.
4. Serve.

Nutrition

Calories: 413 Fat: 1g Carb: 94g Protein: 11g

Strawberry and Chia Seed Overnight Oats Parfait

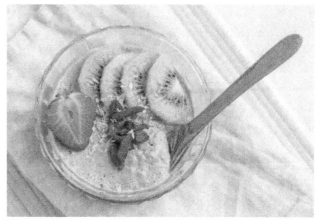

Preparation time: 10 minutes | **Cooking time:** 0 minutes | **Servings:** 2

Ingredients:

For strawberry mixture:

o   1 cup diced strawberries

- o   1 teaspoon chia seeds
- o   1 to 2 teaspoons brown rice syrup
- o   For oat mixture:
- o   1 cup quick rolled oats
- o   1 cup coconut milk (boxed)
- o   1 tablespoon brown rice syrup
- o   ⅛ tablespoon vanilla bean powder

Directions:

Strawberry mixture:

1. In a small bowl, stir together the strawberries, chia seeds, and brown rice syrup until well combined.
2. Oat mixture:
3. In a small bowl, stir together the oats, coconut milk, brown rice syrup, and vanilla bean powder until well combined.
4. Place half the oat mixture in the bottom of 1 large glass mason jar or 2 small jars, and layer half of the strawberry mixture over the oat mixture. Repeat with the remaining oat and strawberry mixtures.
5. Cover the mason jar and refrigerate overnight.
6. Uncover and enjoy.

Nutrition

Calories: 245 kcal Fat: 6g Carbs: 12g Protein: 8g

Carrot and Hemp Seed Muffins

Preparation time: 5 minutes | **Cooking time:** 25 minutes | **Servings:** 12

Ingredients:

- o   3 tablespoons water
- o   1 tablespoon ground flaxseed
- o   2 cups oat flour
- o   1 cup almond milk (boxed)
- o   ½ cup unrefined whole cane sugar
- o   1 carrot, shredded
- o   6 tablespoons cashew butter
- o   2 tablespoons hemp seeds
- o   1 tablespoon chopped lacinato kale
- o   1 tablespoon baking powder
- o   ⅛ teaspoon vanilla bean powder
- o   Pinch sea salt

Directions:

1. Preheat the oven to 350°F.

2. To prepare a flax egg, in a small bowl, whisk together the water and flaxseed.
3. Transfer the flax egg to a medium bowl, and add the oat flour, almond milk, sugar, carrot, cashew butter, hemp seeds, kale, baking powder, vanilla bean powder, and salt, stirring until well combined.
4. Divide the mixture evenly among 12 muffin cups, bake for 20 to 25 minutes, and enjoy right away.

Nutrition

Calories: 334 kcal Fat: 5.6g Carbs: 19.5g Protein: 25.5g

Raspberry-Avocado Smoothie Bowl

Preparation time: 5 minutes | **Cooking time:** 0 minutes | **Servings:** 2

Ingredients:

- o   1½ cups coconut milk (boxed)
- o   1 cup raspberries, plus more (optional) for topping
- o   1 avocado, roughly chopped
- o   3 tablespoons unrefined whole cane sugar
- o   1 teaspoon chia seeds
- o   1 teaspoon unsweetened shredded coconut
- o   Mixed berries, for topping (optional)

Directions:

1. In a blender, blend to combine the coconut milk, raspberries, avocado, and 2 tablespoons of sugar until smooth and creamy.
2. Pour the mixture into 2 serving bowls, sprinkle the extra raspberries (if using), the remaining 1 tablespoon of the sugar, and the chia seeds, shredded coconut, and mixed berries (if using) over the top, and enjoy.

Nutrition

Calories: 145 kcal Fat: 3.5g Carbs: 5.7g Protein: 6.7g

Sweet Potato and Kale Breakfast Hash

Preparation time: 10 minutes | Cooking time: 15 minutes | Servings: 2

Ingredients:

- o   1 teaspoon avocado oil
- o   2 cups peeled and cubed sweet potatoes

o ½ cup chopped kale

o ½ cup diced onion

o ½ teaspoon sea salt

o ½ teaspoon freshly ground black pepper

o ½ avocado, cubed (optional)

o 1 to 2 teaspoons sesame seeds or hemp seeds (optional)

Directions:

1. In a large skillet over medium heat, heat the avocado oil. Add the sweet potatoes, kale, onion, salt, and pepper, and sauté for 10 to 15 minutes, or until the sweet potatoes are soft. Remove from the heat.

2. Gently stir in the avocado and sesame seeds (if using), transfer to 1 large or 2 small plates, and enjoy.

Nutrition

Calories: 176 kcal Fat: 3.3g Carbs: 14.8g Protein: 17.0g

Avocados with Kale and Almond Stuffing

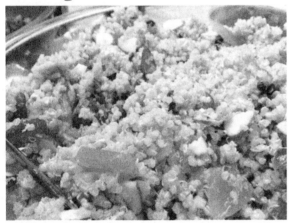

Preparation time: 5 minutes | **Cooking time:** 0 minutes | **Servings:** 2

Ingredients:

o ½ cup almonds

o ½ cup chopped lacinato kale

o 1 garlic clove

o ½ jalapeño

o 2 tablespoons nutritional yeast

o 1 tablespoon avocado oil

o 1 tablespoon apple cider vinegar

o 1 tablespoon freshly squeezed lemon juice

o ¼ teaspoon sea salt

o 1 avocado, halved and pitted

Directions:

1. In a food processor, pulse the almonds, kale, garlic, jalapeño, nutritional yeast, avocado oil, apple cider vinegar, lemon juice, and sea salt until everything is well combined,

2. the almonds are in small pieces, and it has a chunky texture, taking care not to over process.

3. Add half of the stuffing mixture to the center of each avocado half and enjoy.

Nutrition

Calories: 265 kcal Fat: 1.1g Carbs: 15.1g Protein: 19.4g

Mixed Berry–Chia Seed Pudding
Preparation time: 5 minutes | Cooking time: 0 minutes | Servings: 1

Ingredients:

o 1 cup coconut milk (boxed)

o ½ cup mixed berries (raspberries, blackberries, blueberries), plus more (optional) for topping

o 2 tablespoons chia seeds

o 1 to 2 tablespoons unrefined whole cane sugar

Directions:

1. In a mason jar, combine the coconut milk, berries, chia seeds, and sugar, adjusting the sugar to your preference.

2. Seal the jar tightly and shake vigorously until well mixed.

3. Refrigerate for about 1 hour, or until the pudding thickens to your preference.

4. Stir, top with the extra mixed berries, and enjoy.

Nutrition

Calories: 316 kcal Fat: 4.4g Carbs: 10.6g Protein: 16.4g

Pineapple and Coconut Oatmeal Bowl

Preparation time: 5 minutes | **Cooking time:** 5 minutes | **Servings:** 1

Ingredients:

For oatmeal:

o 1 cup quick rolled oats

o 1 (13.5-ounce) can full-fat coconut milk

o 2 tablespoons unrefined whole cane sugar

o   For assembling:

o   ½ cup cubed pineapple

o   ¼ cup unsweetened coconut flakes

o   1 tablespoon chia seeds

o   1 tablespoon pumpkin seeds, chopped

Directions:

For oatmeal:

1.   In a small saucepan over medium-low heat, cook the oats, coconut milk, and sugar for 3 to 5 minutes, or until the oats are soft; adjust the sugar to your preference.

2.   for assemble:

3.   Transfer the oatmeal to 2 serving bowls, top with the cubed pineapple, coconut flakes, and chia and pumpkin seeds, and serve.

Nutrition

Calories: 423 kcal Fat: 3.5g Carbs: 11.6g Protein: 24.8g

Oatmeal Porridge with Mango-Chia Fruit Jam

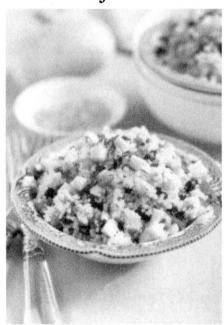

Preparation time: 5 minutes | **Cooking time:** 5 minutes | **Servings:** 2

Ingredients:

o   1 (14-ounce) can full-fat coconut milk

o   1 cup quick rolled oats

o   2 tablespoons unrefined whole cane sugar

o   1 to 2 tablespoons mango Chia Seed Fruit Jam

Directions:

1.   In a small saucepan over medium-low heat, cook the coconut milk, oats, and sugar, stirring occasionally, for 3 to 5 minutes, or until the oats are soft.

2.   Transfer the oatmeal to 2 serving bowls, top with the mango Chia Seed Fruit Jam, and serve.

Nutrition

Calories: 265 kcal Fat: 8.3g Carbs: 13.5g Protein: 16.8g

Vanilla Bean and Cinnamon Granola

Preparation time: 5 minutes | **Cooking time:** 30 minutes | **Servings:** 2

Ingredients:

o   3 cups quick rolled oats

o   ½ cup brown rice syrup

o   6 tablespoons coconut oil

o   ¼ cup unrefined whole cane sugar

o   2 teaspoons vanilla bean powder

o   2 teaspoons ground cinnamon

o   ¼ teaspoon sea salt

Directions:

1.   Preheat the oven to 250°F. Line a baking pan with parchment paper.

2.   In a large bowl, use your hands to mix the oats, brown rice syrup, coconut oil, sugar, vanilla bean powder, cinnamon, and salt until well combined.

3.   Squeeze the mixture together into a ball, and transfer to the prepared baking pan.

4.   Press the mixture evenly on the baking pan, taking care not to break it up into small pieces. This will allow it to bake in large cluster pieces that you can break apart after baking, if you prefer.

5.   Bake for about 30 minutes, or until crispy, taking care not to overbake.

6.   Cool completely before serving. The granola will harden and get even crispier as it cools. Store in an airtight container.

Nutrition

Calories: 366 kcal Fat: 1.4g Carbs: 11.2g Protein: 27.4g

Sesame and Hemp Seed Breakfast Cookies

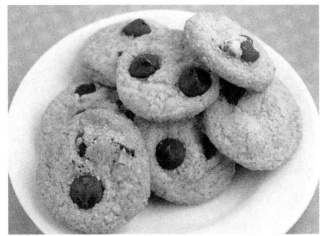

Preparation time: 10 minutes | **Cooking time:** 0 minutes | **Servings:** 15

Ingredients:

o ⅔ cup cashew butter

o ½ cup quick rolled oats

o ¼ cup hemp seeds

o ¼ cup sesame seeds

o 3 tablespoons brown rice syrup

o 3 tablespoons coconut oil, melted

o 1 teaspoon vanilla bean powder

o 1 teaspoon ground cinnamon

Directions:

1. Line a baking sheet with parchment paper.
2. In a medium bowl, stir together the cashew butter, oats, hemp seeds, sesame seeds, brown rice syrup, coconut oil, vanilla bean powder, and cinnamon until well combined.
3. Refrigerate the bowl for 5 to 10 minutes to allow the mixture firm up.
4. Scoop a tablespoonful of dough at a time and flatten into a disk with your hands. Smooth the outer edges with your fingertips, and place on the prepared baking sheet. Repeat with the remaining dough.
5. Refrigerate the cookies for about 20 minutes, or until they firm up, and serve. Store leftovers in an airtight container in the refrigerator; they will soften and lose their shape at room temperature.

Nutrition

Calories: 204 kcal Fat: 4.2g Carbs: 7.3g Protein: 26.3g

Fresh Fruit with Vanilla-Cashew Cream

Preparation time: 25 minutes | **Cooking time:** 0 minutes | **Servings:** 4

Ingredients:

o Room-temperature water, for soaking

o 1 cup raw cashews

o 1 (13.5-ounce) can coconut milk

o 2 tablespoons brown rice syrup

o 2 tablespoons unrefined whole cane sugar

o 2 teaspoons vanilla bean powder

o 1 teaspoon freshly squeezed lemon juice

o ¼ teaspoon ground cinnamon

o ¼ teaspoon sea salt

o 4 cups alkaline fruit, such as raspberries, blackberries, blueberries, strawberries, mango, pineapple, or cantaloupe

Directions:

1. In a medium bowl with enough room-temperature water to cover them, soak the cashews for 15 to 20 minutes.
2. Drain and rinse the cashews.
3. In a high-speed blender, blend to combine the soaked cashews, coconut milk, brown rice syrup, sugar, vanilla bean powder, lemon juice, cinnamon, and salt until creamy and smooth. Add more sugar if you like.
4. Add 1 cup of fruit to each of 4 serving bowls, drizzle each bowl of fruit with ½ cup of cream, and serve.

Nutrition

Calories: 346 kcal Fat: 5.8g Carbs: 15.4g Protein: 17.2g

Pumpkin Seed–Protein Breakfast Balls

Preparation time: 5 minutes | **Cooking time:** 0 minutes | **Servings:** 20

Ingredients:

o 1½ cups quick rolled oats

o 3 tablespoons 100% organic pumpkin seed protein powder

o ½ cup almond butter

o ½ cup raw pumpkin seeds

o 3 tablespoons brown rice syrup

o   1 tablespoon coconut oil

o   1 teaspoon ground cinnamon

o   1 teaspoon vanilla bean powder

o   2 to 4 tablespoons coconut milk

Directions:

1.   Line a baking sheet with parchment paper.

2.   In a food processor, process the oats, protein powder, almond butter, pumpkin seeds, brown rice syrup, coconut oil, cinnamon, vanilla bean powder, and coconut milk until well combined, taking care to not over process.

3.   Scoop a tablespoonful into your hands and roll into a ball. Place on the prepared baking sheet and repeat with the remaining mixture.

4.   Refrigerate for 15 to 20 minutes, or until firm, and serve. Store in the refrigerator; the balls will get soft and lose their shape at room temperature.

Nutrition

Calories: 198 kcal Fat: 3.7g Carbs: 13.4g Protein: 16g

No-Bake Granola Bars

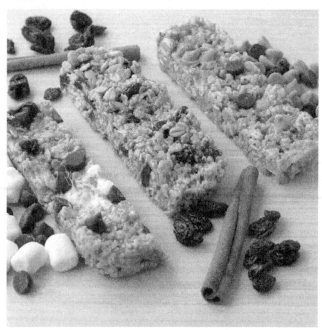

Preparation time: 5 minutes | **Cooking:** 0 minutes

Servings: 5

Ingredients:

o   1 cup quick rolled oats

o   ½ cup almond butter

o   2 tablespoons brown rice syrup

o   1 tablespoon coconut oil

o   ¼ teaspoon sea salt

o   ¼ teaspoon ground cinnamon

o   ¼ teaspoon vanilla bean powder

Directions:

1.   Line a 9-by-5-inch loaf dish with parchment paper.

2.   In a food processor, process the oats, almond butter, brown rice syrup, coconut oil, salt, cinnamon, and vanilla bean powder until well combined.

3.   Transfer the mixture to the prepared loaf dish and press down firmly and evenly with your hand and fingertips.

4.   Refrigerate for 15 to 20 minutes, or until the mixture firms up.

5.   Cut into 6 bars or 12 squares and serve. Store in the refrigerator; the bars will get soft and lose their shape at room temperature.

Nutrition

Calories: 256 kcal Fat: 6g Carbs: 13g Protein: 20g

Smoothie

Nori Clove Smoothies (NCS)

Preparation Time: 10 minutes | **Cooking Time:** 0 minutes | **Servings:** 1

Ingredients:

o ¼ cup fresh nori

o 1 cup cubed banana

o 1 teaspoon diced onion or ¼ teaspoon powdered onion

o ½ teaspoon clove

o 1 cup Dr. Sebi's energy booster

o 1 tablespoon agave syrup

Directions:

1. Rinse ANCS Items with clean water.
2. Finely chop the onion to take one teaspoon and cut fresh nori.
3. Boil 1½ teaspoon with 2 cups of water, remove the particle, allow to cool, measure 1 cup of the tea extract.
4. Pour all the items inside a blender with the tea extract and blend to achieve homogenous smoothies.
5. Transfer into a clean cup and have a nice time with a lovely body detox and energizer.

Nutrition

Calories: 78 Fat: 2.3 g Carb: 5 g Protein: 6 g

Brazil Lettuce Smoothies (BLS)

Preparation Time: 10 minutes | **Cooking Time:** 0 minutes | **Servings:** 1

Ingredients:

o 1 cup raspberries

o ½ handful Romaine lettuce

o ½ cup homemade walnut milk

o 2 Brazil nuts

o ½ large grape with seed

o 1 cup soft jelly coconut water

o Date Sugar to Taste

Directions:

1. In a clean bowl rinse, the fruits with clean water.
2. Chop the Romaine lettuce and cubed raspberries and add other items into the blender and blend to achieve homogenous smoothies.
3. Serve your delicious medicinal detox.

Nutrition

Calories: 168 Fat: 4.5 g Carbohydrates: 31.3 g Sugar: 19.2 g Protein: 3.6 g

Apple – Banana Smoothie (ABS)

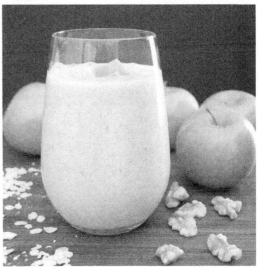

Preparation Time: 10 minutes | **Cooking Time:** 0 minutes | **Servings:** 1

Ingredients:

o 1 cup cubed apple

o ½ burro banana

o ½ cup cubed mango

o ½ cup cubed watermelon

o ½ teaspoon powdered onion

o 3 tablespoon Key lime juice

o Date sugar to taste (If you like)

Directions:

1. In a clean bowl rinse, the fruits with clean water.
2. Add cubed banana, apple, mango, watermelon, and add other items into the blender and blend to achieve homogenous smoothies.
3. Serve your delicious medicinal detox.
4. Alternatively, you can add one tablespoon of finely dices raw red onion if the powdered onion is not available.

Nutrition

Calories: 99 Fat: 0.3g Carb: 23 g Protein: 1.1 g

Ginger – Pear Smoothie (GPS)

Preparation Time: 10 minutes | **Cooking Time:** 0 minutes | **Servings:** 1

Ingredients:

o 1 big pear with seed and cured

o ½ avocado

o ¼ handful watercress

o ½ sour orange

o ½ cup of ginger tea

o ½ cup of coconut water

o ¼ cup of spring water

o 2 tablespoons agave syrup

o Date sugar to satisfaction

Directions:

1. Firstly, boil 1 cup of ginger tea, cover the cup, and allow it cool to room temperature.
2. Pour all the AGPS Items into your clean blender and homogenize them to smooth fluid.
3. You have just prepared yourself a wonderful detox Romaine smoothie.

Nutrition

Calories : 101 Protein : 1 g Crabs : 27 g Fiber : 6 g

Cantaloupe – Amaranth Smoothie

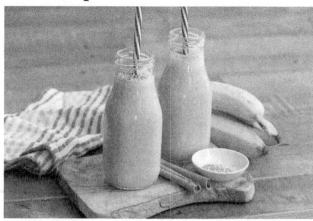

Preparation Time: 10 minutes | **Cooking Time:** 0 minutes | **Servings:** 1

Ingredients:

o ½ cup of cubed cantaloupe

o ¼ handful green amaranth

o ½ cup homemade hemp milk

o ¼ teaspoon Dr. Sebi's bromide plus powder

o 1 cup of coconut water

o 1 teaspoon agave syrup

Directions:

1. You will have to rinse all the ACAS items with clean water.
2. Chop green amaranth, cubed cantaloupe, transfer all into a blender and blend to achieve a homogenous smoothie.
3. Pour into a clean cup; add Agave syrup and homemade hemp milk.
4. Stir them together and drink.

Nutrition

Calories : 55 Fiber : 1.5 g Carbohydrates : 8 g Proteins 2g

Garbanzo Squash Smoothie (GSS)

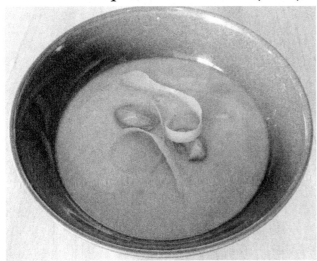

Preparation Time: 10 minutes | **Cooking Time:** 0 minutes | **Servings:** 1

Ingredients:

o 1 large, cubed apple

o 1 fresh tomato

o 1 tablespoon finely chopped fresh onion or ¼ teaspoon powdered onion

o ¼ cup boiled garbanzo bean

o ½ cup of coconut milk

o ¼ cubed Mexican squash chayote

o 1 cup energy booster tea

Directions:

1. You will need to rinse the AGSS items with clean water.

2. Boil 1½ Dr. Sebi's energy booster tea with 2 cups of clean water. Filter the extract, measure 1 cup, and allow it to cool.

3. Cook Garbanzo beans, drain the water and allow it to cool.

4. Pour all the AGSS items into a high-speed blender and blend to achieve a homogenous smoothie.

5. You may add date sugar.

6. Serve your amazing smoothie and drink.

Nutrition

Calories: 82 Carbs: 22 g Protein: 2 g Fiber: 7 g

Strawberry – Orange Smoothies

Preparation Time: 10 minutes | **Cooking Time:** 0 minutes | **Servings:** 1

Ingredients:

o 1 cup of diced strawberries

o 1 removed back of Seville orange

o ¼ cup cubed cucumber

o ¼ cup Romaine lettuce

o ½ kelp

o ½ burro banana

o 1 cup soft jelly coconut water

o ½ cup of water

o Date sugar

Directions:

1. Use clean water to rinse all the vegetable items of ASOS into a clean bowl.

2. Chop Romaine lettuce; dice strawberry, cucumber, and banana; remove the back of Seville orange and divide into four.

3. Transfer all the ASOS items inside a clean blender and blend to achieve a homogenous smoothie.

4. Pour into a clean big cup and fortify your body with a palatable detox.

Nutrition

Calories 298 Calories from Fat 9 Fat 1g Cholesterol 2mg Sodium 73mg Potassium 998mg Carbohydrates 68g Fiber 7g Sugar 50g

Tamarind – Pear Smoothie (TPS)

Preparation Time: 10 minutes | **Cooking Time:** 0 minutes | **Servings:** 1

Ingredients:

o ½ burro banana

o ½ cup of watermelon

o 1 raspberry

o 1 prickly pear

o 1 grape with seed

o 3 tamarinds

o ½ medium cucumber

o 1 cup of coconut water

o ½ cup Distilled water

Directions:

1. Use clean water to rinse all the ATPS items.
2. Remove the pod of tamarinds and collect the edible part around the seed into a container.
3. If you must use the seeds, then you must boil the seed for 15 minutes and add to the tamarind edible part in the container.
4. Cube all other vegetable fruits and transfer all the items into a high-speed blender and blend to achieve a homogenous smoothie.

Nutritions

Calories: 199 Carbs: 47g Fats: 1g Proteins: 6g

Currant Elderberry Smoothie

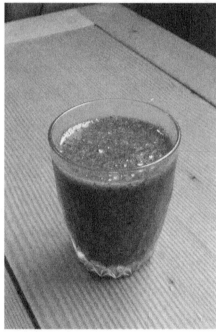

Preparation Time: 10 minutes | **Cooking Time:** 0 minutes | **Servings:** 1

Ingredients:

o ¼ cup cubed elderberry

o 1 sour cherry

o 2 currants

o 1 cubed burro banana

o 1 fig

o 1 cup 4 bay leaves tea

o 1 cup energy booster tea

o Date sugar to your satisfaction

Directions:

1. Use clean water to rinse all the ACES items.
2. Initially boil ¾ teaspoon of energy Booster Tea with 2 cups of water on a heat source and allow boiling for 10 minutes.
3. Add 4 bay leaves and boil together for another 4 minutes.
4. Drain the tea extract into a clean big cup and allow it to cool.
5. Transfer all the items into a high-speed blender and blend till you achieve a homogenous smoothie.
6. Pour the palatable medicinal smoothie into a clean cup and drink.

Nutrition

Calories: 63 Fat: 0.22g Sodium: 1.1mg Carbs: 15.5g Fiber: 4.8g Sugars: 8.25g Protein:1.6g

Sweet Dream Strawberry Smoothie

Preparation Time: 15 minutes | **Cooking Time:** 0 | **Servings:** 1

Ingredients:

o 5 strawberries

o 3 dates – pits eliminated

o 2 burro bananas or small bananas

o Spring water for 32 fluid ounces of smoothie

Directions:

1. Strip off the skin of the bananas.
2. Wash the dates and strawberries.
3. Include bananas, dates, and strawberries to a blender container.
4. Include a couple of water and blend.
5. Keep on including adequate water to persuade up to be 32 oz. of smoothie.

Nutrition

Calories: 282 Fat: 11g Carb: 4g Protein: 7g

Alkaline Green Ginger and Banana Cleansing Smoothie

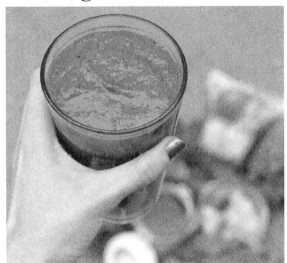

Preparation Time: 15 minutes | **Cooking Time:** 0 | **Servings:** 1

Ingredients:

o   One handful of kale
o   One banana, frozen
o   Two cups of hemp seed milk
o   One inch of ginger, finely minced
o   Half cup of chopped strawberries, frozen
o   1 tablespoon of agave or your preferred sweetener

Directions:

1. Mix all the ingredients in a blender and mix on high speed.
2. Allow it to blend evenly.
3. Pour into a pitcher with a few decorative straws and voila, you are one happy camper.
4. Enjoy!

Nutrition

Calories: 350 Fat: 4g Carb: 52g Protein: 16g

Orange Mixed Detox Smoothie

Preparation Time: 15 minutes | **Cooking Time:** 0 | **Servings:** 1

Ingredients:

o   One cup of veggies (amaranth, dandelion, lettuce, or watercress)
o   Half avocado
o   One cup of tender-jelly coconut water
o   One Seville orange
o   Juice of one key lime
o   One tablespoon of bromide plus powder

Directions:

1. Peel and cut the Seville orange in chunks.
2. Mix all the ingredients collectively in a high-speed blender until done.

Nutrition

Calories: 71 Fat: 1g Carbohydrates: 12g Protein: 2g

Cucumber Toxin Flush Smoothie

Preparation Time: 15 minutes | **Cooking Time:** 0 | **Servings:** 1

Ingredients:

o   1 cucumber
o   1 key lime
o   1 cup of watermelon (seeded), cubed

Directions:

1. Mix all the above ingredients in a high-speed blender.
2. Considering that watermelon and cucumbers are largely water, you may not want to add any extra, however, you can do so if you want.
3. Juice the key lime and add it to your smoothie.
4. Enjoy!

Nutrition

Calories: 219 Fat: 4g Carb: 48g Protein: 5g

Apple Blueberry Smoothie

Preparation Time: 15 minutes | **Cooking Time:** 0 | **Servings:** 1

Ingredients:

o   Half apple
o   One date
o   Half cup of blueberries
o   Half cup of sparkling callaloo
o   One tablespoon of hemp seeds

o   One tablespoon of sesame seeds

o   Two cups of sparkling soft-jelly coconut water

o   Half tablespoon of bromide plus powder

Directions:

1.   Mix all the ingredients in a high-speed blender

2.   Enjoy!

Nutrition

Calories: 167.4 Fat: 6.4g Carbohydrates: 22.5g Protein: 6.7g

Detox Berry Smoothie

Preparation Time: 15 minutes | **Cooking Time:** 0 | **Servings:** 1

Ingredients:

o   Spring water

o   1/4 avocado, pitted

o   One medium burro banana

o   One Seville orange

o   Two cups of fresh lettuce

o   One tablespoon of hemp seeds

o   One cup of berries (blueberries or an aggregate of blueberries, strawberries, and raspberries)

Directions:

1.   Add the spring water to your blender.

2.   Put the fruits and veggies right inside the blender.

3.   Blend all ingredients until smooth.

Nutrition

Calories: 202.4   Fat: 4.5g Carbs: 32.9g Proteins: 13.3g

Papaya Detox Smoothie

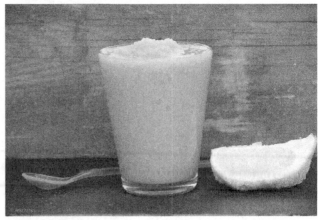

Preparation Time: 15 minutes | **Cooking Time:** 0 | **Servings:** 1

Ingredients:

o   Two cups papaya

o   One tablespoon of papaya seeds

o   Juice of a Lime

o   One cup of filtered water

Directions:

1.   Chop the papaya into square portions and scoop out a tablespoon of clean and raw papaya seeds.

2.   Mix all the ingredients right into a high-speed blender for 1 minute until the whole thing is blended.

3.   Pour into a tumbler and enjoy this tasty drink your liver will love.

4.   Enjoy!

Nutrition

Calories: 197 Fat: 0.7g Carb: 49.4g Protein: 5.4g

Apple and Amaranth Detoxifying Smoothie

Preparation Time: 15 minutes | **Cooking Time:** 0 | **Servings:** 1

Ingredients:

o   1/4 avocado

o   1 key lime

o   Two apples, chopped

o   Two cups of water

o   Two cups of amaranth veggie

Directions:

1. Put all the ingredients collectively in a blender.
2. Blend all the ingredients evenly.
3. Enjoy this delicious smoothie.

Nutrition

Calories: 133 Fats: 4g Carbs: 24g Proteins: 3g

Avocado Mixed Smoothie

Preparation Time: 15 minutes | **Cooking Time:** 0 | **Servings.** 1

Ingredients:

o One cup of water
o One ounce of blueberries
o One pear, chopped
o 1/4 avocado, pitted
o 1/4 cup cooked quinoa

Directions:

1. Mix all ingredients in a high-speed blender
2. Enjoy!

Nutrition

Calories: 187 Fat: 21g Carb: 29g Protein: 11g

Peach Berry Smoothie

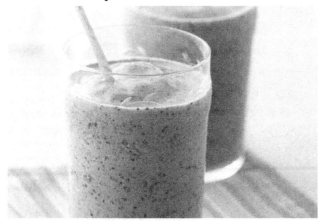

Preparation Time: 15 minutes | **Cooking Time:** 0 | **Servings:** 1

Ingredients:

o Half cup of frozen peaches
o Half cup of frozen blueberries
o Half cup of frozen cherries
o Half cup of frozen strawberries

o One tablespoon of sea moss gel
o One tablespoon of hemp seeds
o One tablespoon of coconut water
o One tablespoon of agave

Directions:

1. Blend all ingredients for one minute.
2. If the combination is too thick, add extra ¼ cup of coconut water and blend for another 20 secs.
3. Enjoy your peach berry smoothie!

Nutrition

Calories: 170 Fat: 0g Carbohydrates: 43g

Irish Sea Moss Smoothie

Preparation Time: 15 minutes | **Cooking Time:** 0 | **Servings:** 1

Ingredients:

o 2 oz. of whole wild sea moss, soaked
o 2 cups of spring water

Directions:

1. To prepare Irish sea moss smoothie, use two whole and wild sea moss.
2. Carefully wash away any sand and debris.
3. Do a final wash and chop up longer ones to safeguard your blender's blade.
4. Add your sea moss and two cups of spring water to blend in the blender.
5. Put in a jar and refrigerate. This smoothie can last for many weeks.
6. Enjoy your delicious smoothie.

Nutrition

Calories: 220 Fat: 3g Carb: 45g Protein: 2g

Cucumber Mixed Detox Smoothie

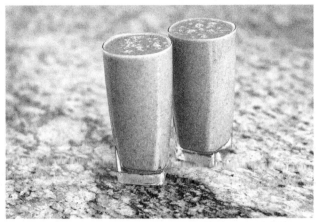

Preparation Time: 15 minutes | **Cooking Time:** 0 | **Servings:** 1

Ingredients:

o   Half cucumber, chopped

o   One inch of ginger

o   One pinch of pure sea salt

o   Two grapefruits, squeezed

o   Two lemons, squeezed

o   One avocado, chopped

o   Half cup of filtered or spring water

o   One pinch cayenne pepper

Directions:

1.   Blend all ingredients.

2.   Sip and experience this tasty nutritious smoothie!

Nutrition

Calories: 48 Fat: 0g Carbohydrates: 12g Protein: 1g

Strawberry Banana Smoothie

Preparation Time: 15 minutes | **Cooking Time:** 0 | **Servings:** 1-2

Ingredients:

o   2 cups hemp milk

o   4 bananas

o   8 oz. strawberry

o   ¾ cup dates

o   1 tbsp. agave

Directions:

1.   To make this delicious smoothie, you need to place the strawberries and date in a high-speed blender.

2.   Blend them for a minute or two or until they are slightly broken down.

3.   After that, add the banana along with the hemp milk and agave.

4.   Blend them for 2 to 3 minutes or until combined well.

5.   Enjoy.

Nutrition

Calories: 148 Fat: 2g Carb: 21g Protein: 1g

Green Monster Smoothie

Preparation Time: 15 minutes | **Cooking Time:** 0 | **Servings:** 1

Ingredients:

o   ½ of 1 avocado, diced

o   ½ of 1 mango, diced

o   2 to 3 dates, pitted

o   1 tbsp. soursop pulp

o   1 bunch of rainbow Kale, leaves torn

o   ½ cup of coconut water

Directions:

1.   To make this smoothie, place all the ingredients in a high-speed blender and blend it for 2 to 3 minutes or until everything comes together and smooth.

2.   Move the mixture to a serving glass and serve it with ice cubes if you desire to take it cold.

Nutrition

Calories: 179.4 Fat: 2.3g Carbohydrates: 36.8g Protein: 6.8g

Apple Smoothie

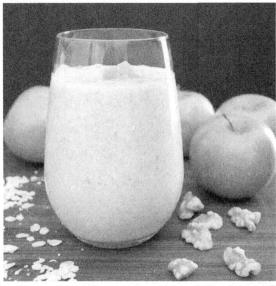

Preparation Time: 15 minutes | **Cooking Time:** 0 | **Servings:** 2

Ingredients:

o 2 cups of apple juice, fresh

o 2 cups ice cube

o 1 tbsp. sea moss

o 1 clove, grounded

o 1 tbsp. ginger, grounded

Directions:

1. To start with, place all the ingredients needed to make the smoothie in a high-speed blender.
2. Blend all ingredients wait for 2 to 3 minutes or until you get a smooth mixture.
3. Serve and enjoy.

Nutrition

Calories: 431.5 Fats: 10.8g Carbs: 53.1g Proteins: 38.4g

Weight Loss Apple Cucumber Smoothie

Preparation Time: 15 minutes | **Cooking Time:** 0 | **Servings:** 1

Ingredients:

o One large to medium size of sliced cucumber

o One large, cubed apple

o One large, sliced bell pepper

o Six seeded dates (rinsed)

o Six large strawberries

o Five sliced tomatoes (rinsed)

o Half to one cupful of water

Directions:

1. Combine the whole recipes and blend very well until smooth.
2. Wow! The first-day breakfast is settled, enjoy.

Nutrition

Calories 65 Carb 57 g Protein 2 g Fat 4 g

Toxins Removal Smoothie

Preparation Time: 15 minutes | **Cooking Time:** 0 | **Servings:** 1

Ingredients:

o One seeded and sliced small to large-sized watermelon

o One large key lime (removes the juice and discards the seed

o One large cucumber (sliced)

Directions:

1. Transfer the lime juice into the blender.
2. Add the remaining recipes and blend very well to obtain a smooth mixture.
3. Wow! This means you have successfully completed the second-day smoothie.
4. Enjoy.

Nutrition

Calories 45 Carb 35 g Protein 6 g Fat 4 g

Multiple Berries Smoothie

Preparation Time: 15 minutes | **Cooking Time:** 0 | **Servings:** 1

Ingredients:

o A quarter cupful of blueberries

o A quarter cupful of strawberries

o A quarter cupful of raspberries

o One large banana (peeled and sliced)

o Agave syrup as desired

o A half cupful of water

Directions:

1. Transfer the water into the blender.
2. Add the remaining recipes and blend until smooth.
3. I really love this smoothie because it is very sweet without adding sugar and the color is also inviting.

Nutrition

Calories: 210 Carbohydrates : 55 g Sodium : 20 mg

Dandelion Avocado Smoothie

Preparation Time: 15 minutes | **Cooking Time:** 0 | **Servings:** 1

Ingredients:

o   One cup of dandelion

o   One orange (juiced)

o   Coconut water

o   One avocado

o   One key lime (juice)

Directions:

1. In a high-speed blend all ingredients until smooth.

Nutrition

Calories: 160 Fat: 15 g Carb: 9 g Protein: 2 grams

Amaranth Greens and Avocado Smoothie

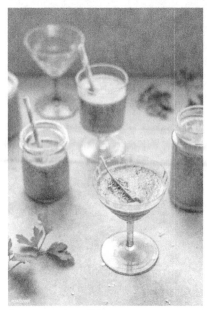

Preparation Time: 15 minutes | **Cooking Time:** 0 | **Servings:** 1

Ingredients:

o   One key lime (juice)

o   Two sliced apples (seeded)

o   Half avocado

o   Two cups of amaranth greens

o   Two cups of watercress

o   One cup of water

Directions:

1. Add the whole recipes together and transfer them into the blender.
2. Blend thoroughly until smooth.

Nutrition

Calories: 160 Fat: 15 g Carb: 9 g Protein: 2 g

Lettuce, Orange, and Banana Smoothie

Preparation Time: 15 minutes | **Cooking Time:** 0 | **Servings:** 1

Ingredients:

o   One and a half cupsful of fresh lettuce

o   One large banana

o   One cup of mixed berries of your choice

o   One juiced orange

Directions:

1.   First, add the orange juice to your blender.
2.   Add the remaining recipes and blend thoroughly.
3.   Enjoy the rest of your day.

Nutrition

Calories: 252.1 Protein: 4.1g Carbs 6g

Delicious Elderberry Smoothie

Preparation Time: 15 minutes | **Cooking Time:** 0 | **Servings:** 1

Ingredients:

o   One cupful of elderberry

o   One cupful of cucumber

o   One large apple

o   A quarter cupful of water

Directions:

1.   Add the whole recipes together into a blender.
2.   Grind very well until they are uniformly smooth and enjoy.

Nutrition

Calories: 106 Carbs: 26g Proteins 4 Fats 1g

Peaches Zucchini Smoothie

Preparation Time: 15 minutes | **Cooking Time:** 0 | **Servings:** 1

Ingredients:

o   A half cupful of squash

o   A half cupful of peaches

o   A quarter cupful of coconut water

o   A half cupful of Zucchini

Directions:

1.   Add the whole recipes together into a blender
2.   blend until smooth and serve.

Nutrition

Calories 55 Fat 0g Protein 2g Sodium 10 mg Carbohydrate 14g   Fiber 2g

Ginger Orange and Strawberry Smoothie

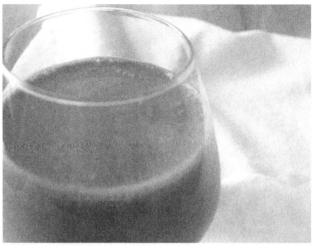

Preparation Time: 15 minutes | **Cooking Time:** 0 | **Servings:** 1

Ingredients:

o   One cup of strawberry

o   One large orange (juice)

o   One large banana

o   Quarter small sized ginger (peeled and sliced)

Directions:

1.   Transfer the orange juice to a clean blender.
2.   Add the remaining recipes and blend thoroughly until smooth.
3.   Enjoy. Wow! You have ended the 9th day of your weight loss and detox journey.

Nutrition

Calories 32 Fat 0.3g Protein 2g Sodium 10mg Carbohydrate 14g Fiber 2g

Kale Parsley and Chia Seeds Detox Smoothie

Preparation Time: 15 minutes | **Cooking Time:** 0 | **Servings:** 1

Ingredients:

o   Three tbsp. chia seeds (grounded)

o   One cupful of water

o   One sliced banana

o   One pear (chopped)

o   One cupful of organic kale

o   One cupful of parsley

o   Two tbsp. of lemon juice

o   A dash of cinnamon

Directions:

1. Add the whole recipes together into a blender and pour the water before blending.

2. Blend at high speed until smooth and enjoy. You may or may not place it in the refrigerator, depending on how hot or cold the weather appears.

Nutrition

Calories 75 Fat 1g Protein 5g Fiber 10g

Herbal Tea Recipes

Chamomile Herbal Tea

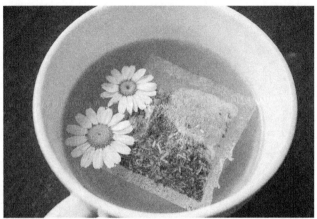

Preparation time: 5 minutes | **Cooking time:** 5 minutes | **Servings:** 2

Ingredients:

o   2 thin apple slices

o   2 cups boiling spring water

o   2 tablespoons fresh chamomile flowers, rinsed

o   1–2 teaspoons agave nectar

Directions:

1.   Rinse the teapot with boiling water.
2.   In the warm pot, place the apple slices and with a wooden spoon, mash them.
3.   Add the chamomile flowers and top with the boiling water.
4.   Cover the pot and steep for 3–5 minutes.
5.   Strain the tea into two serving cups and stir in the agave nectar.
6.   Serve immediately.

Nutrition

Calories 68 Total Fat 0.2 g Saturated Fat 0g Cholesterol 0 mg Sodium 1 mg Total Carbs 18.1 g Fiber 2.9 g Sugar 14.1 g Protein 0.3 g

Burdock Herbal Tea

Preparation time: 5 minutes | **Cooking time:** 5 minutes | **Servings:** 2

Ingredients:

o   2 teaspoons dried burdock root

o   2 cups boiling spring water

Directions:

1.   In a teapot, add the burdock root and top with the boiling water.
2.   Cover the pot and steep for 3–5 minutes.
3.   Strain the tea into two serving cups and serve immediately.

Nutrition

Calories 2 Total Fat 0 g Saturated Fat 0 g Cholesterol 0 mg Sodium 0 mg Total Carbs 0.4 g Fiber 0.1g Sugar 0.1 g Protein 0 g

Elderberry Herbal Tea

Preparation time: 10 minutes | **Cooking time:** 20 minutes | **Servings:** 2

Ingredients:

o   16 ounces spring water

o   2 tablespoons dried elderberries

o   ½ teaspoon ground turmeric

o   ¼ teaspoon ground cinnamon

o   1 teaspoon agave nectar

Directions:

1.   In a small saucepan, place water and elderberries, turmeric and cinnamon over medium-high heat and bring to a boil.
2.   Now, adjust the heat to low and simmer for about 15 minutes.
3.   Remove from heat and set aside to cool for about 5 minutes.
4.   Through a fine mesh strainer, strain the tea into serving cups and stir in the agave nectar.
5.   Serve immediately.

Nutrition

Calories 19 Total Fat 0.1 g Saturated Fat 0 g Cholesterol 0 mg Sodium 1 mg Total Carbs 4.9 g Fiber 1.1 g Sugar 2.5 g Protein 0.1 g

Fennell Herbal Tea

Preparation time: 5 minutes | **Cooking time:** 5 minutes | **Servings:** 2

Ingredients:

o   2–4 teaspoons fennel seeds, crushed freshly

o   2 cups boiling spring water

Directions:

1.   In a teapot, add the fennel seeds and top with the boiling water.
2.   Cover the pot and steep for 5–10 minutes.
3.   Strain the tea into two serving cups and serve immediately.

Nutrition

Calories 7 Total Fat 0.3 g Saturated Fat 0 g Cholesterol 0 mg Sodium 2 mg Total Carbs 1.1g Fiber 0.8 g Sugar 0 g Protein 0.3 g

Fennel & Ginger Herbal Tea

Preparation time: 10 minutes | **Cooking time:** 5 minutes | **Servings:** 2

Ingredients:

o   2 cups spring water

o   1 tablespoon fennel seeds, crushed slightly

o   1 (½-inch) piece fresh ginger, peeled and crushed slightly

o   2 teaspoons agave nectar

Directions:

1.   In a small saucepan, add water over medium heat and bring to a rolling boil.
2.   Stir in the fennel seeds and ginger and remove from the heat.
3.   Strain the tea into two serving cups and stir in the agave nectar.
4.   Serve immediately.

Nutrition

Calories 33 Total Fat 0.5 g Saturated Fat 0 g

Cholesterol 0 mg Sodium 3 mg Total Carbs 7.5 g Fiber 1.6 g Sugar 5 g Protein 0.5 g

Ginger & Cinnamon Herbal Tea

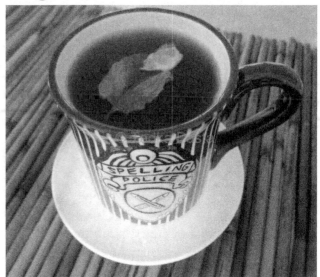

Preparation time: 10 minutes | **Cooking time:** 10 minutes | **Servings:** 1

Ingredients:

o   1 cup spring water

o   1 (1-inch) piece fresh ginger, cut into pieces

o   1 cinnamon stick

o   1 teaspoon agave nectar

Directions:

1.   In a saucepan, add water, ginger, and cinnamon over high heat and bring to a boil.
2.   Now, adjust the heat to low and simmer for about 5 minutes.
3.   Remove the saucepan of tea from the and strain into a serving cup.
4.   Stir in the agave nectar and serve immediately.

Nutrition

Calories 40 Total Fat 0.3 g Saturated Fat 0.1 g Cholesterol 0 mg Sodium 2 mg Total Carbs 9.6 g Fiber 1.3 g Sugar 5.2 g Protein 0.5 g

Ginger & Lime Herbal Tea

Preparation time: 10 minutes | **Cooking time:** 15 minutes | **Servings:** 2

Ingredients:

- o   2 cups spring water
- o   2 tablespoons fresh ginger root, cut into slices
- o   1 tablespoon fresh key lime juice
- o   1 tablespoon agave nectar

Directions:

1. In a saucepan, add water, ginger, and cinnamon over high heat and bring to a boil.
2. Now, adjust the heat to low and simmer for about 10 minutes.
3. Remove the saucepan of tea from the and strain into serving cups.
4. In the cups, stir in the lime juice and agave nectar and serve immediately.

Nutrition

Calories 34 Total Fat 0.1 g Saturated Fat 0 g Cholesterol 0 mg Sodium 0 mg Total Carbs 8.6 g Fiber 0.6 g Sugar 7.6 g Protein 0.1 g

Linden Herbal Tea

Preparation time: 5 minutes | **Cooking time:** 6 minutes | **Servings:** 1

Ingredients:

- o   2 teaspoon fresh linden flowers
- o   1 cup spring water
- o   1 teaspoon agave nectar

Directions:

1. In a saucepan, add water over medium heat and bring to a boil.
2. Stir in the linden flowers and cook for about 1 minute.
3. Remove from the heat and set aside, covered for about 10 minutes.
4. Strain the tea into a serving cup and stir in the agave nectar.
5. Serve immediately.

Nutrition

Calories 20 Total Fat 0 g Saturated Fat 0 g Cholesterol 0 mg Sodium 0 mg Total Carbs 5.3 g Fiber 0.3 g Sugar 5 g Protein 0 g

Raspberry Herbal Tea

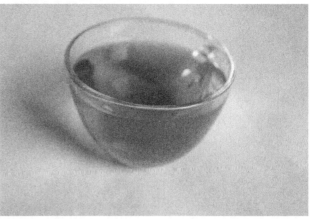

Preparation time: 5 minutes | **Cooking time:** 5 minutes | **Servings:** 1

Ingredients:

- o   1–2 teaspoons red raspberry leaf tea
- o   1 cup boiling spring water
- o   1 teaspoon agave nectar

Directions:

1. In the teapot, place the raspberry leaf tea and top with the boiling water.
2. Cover the pot and steep for 3–5 minutes.
3. Strain the tea into two serving cups and stir in the agave nectar.
4. Serve immediately.

Nutrition

Calories 20   Total Fat 0 g Saturated Fat 0 g Cholesterol 0 mg Sodium 0 mg Total Carbs 5.3 g Fiber 0.3 g Sugar 5 g Protein 0 g

Anise & Cinnamon Herbal Tea

Preparation time: 5 minutes | **Cooking time:** 15 minutes | **Servings:** 2

Ingredients:

- o   7-star anise
- o   1 (2-inch) cinnamon stick
- o   2–3 cups water

Directions:

1. In a saucepan, add water over medium heat and bring to a rolling boil.
2. Add star anise and cinnamon stick and boil for about 10 minutes.

3. Remove from heat and steep, covered for about 3 minutes.
4. Strain the tea into two serving cups and stir in the agave nectar.
5. Serve immediately.

Nutrition

Calories 20 Total Fat 0.6 g Saturated Fat 0 g
Cholesterol 0 mg Sodium 1 mg Total Carbs 4.4 g
Fiber 2.3 g   Sugar 0.1 g   Protein 0 7 g

Salad recipes

Dandelion Strawberry Salad

Preparation Time: 15 minutes | **Cooking Time**: 10 minutes | **Servings**: 2

Ingredients:

o   2 tbsp. grapeseed oil

o   1 medium red onion, sliced

o   10 ripe strawberries, sliced

o   2 tbsp. key lime juice

o   4 cups dandelion greens

o   Sea salt to taste

Directions:

1.   First of all, warm grapeseed oil in a 12-inch non-stick frying pan over medium heat. Add some sliced onions and a small pinch of sea salt. Cook until the onions are soft, lightly brown, and reduced to about 1/3 of raw volume, stirring frequently.

2.   Then toss strawberry slices in a tiny bowl with 1 teaspoon of key lime juice. Rinse the dandelion greens and, if you prefer, slice them into chunks of bite-size.

3.   When it's about to be cooked, put the remaining key lime juice to the saucepan and keep on cooking until it has thickened to coat the onions for a minute or two. Remove the onions from heat.

4.   Combine the vegetables, onions, and strawberries with all their juices in a salad bowl. Sprinkle with sea salt.

Nutrition

Calories: 151 Carbs: 2g Fats: 13g Proteins: 7g

Headache Preventing Salad

Preparation Time: 5 minutes | **Cooking Time**: 0 minutes | **Servings**: 1

Ingredients:

o   1/2 seeded cucumber

o   2 cups watercress

o   2 tbsp. olive oil

o   1 tbsp key lime juice

o   Salt and cayenne pepper, to taste

Directions:

1.   Combine with the olive oil and key lime until well blended. Arrange the watercress and cucumber.

2.   Add the dressing to taste, then sprinkle with salt and pepper. Serve.

Nutrition

Calories: 52 Carbs: 12g Fat: 0g Protein: 1g

Detox Watercress Citrus Salad

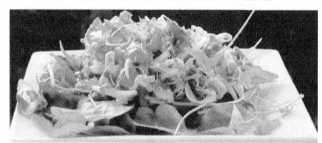

Preparation Time: 5 minutes | **Cooking Time**: 0 minutes | **Servings**: 1

Ingredients:

o   1 avocado, ripe

o   4 cups watercress

o   1 Seville orange, zested, peeled, and sliced

o   2 skinny slices of red onion

o   2 tsp. agave syrup

o   2 tbsp. Key lime juice

o   2 tbsp. olive oil

o   1/8 tsp. salt

o   Cayenne pepper, optional

Directions:

1.   Set on two plates watercress, avocado, onion, and oranges.

2.   In a small bowl, mix the key lime juice, olive oil, agave syrup, salt, and cayenne pepper. When

ready to be served, spoon the dressing over the salad.

Nutrition

Calories: 130 Carbs: 23g Fat: 3g Protein: 3g

Basil Avocado Pasta Salad

Preparation Time: 5 minutes | **Cooking Time**: 0 minutes | **Servings**: 1

Ingredients:

o   1 avocado, chopped

o   1 cup fresh basil, chopped

o   1-pint cherry tomatoes halved

o   1 tbsp. key lime juice

o   1 tsp. agave syrup

o   1/4 cup olive oil

o   4 cups cooked spelt-pasta

Directions:

1.   Place the cooked pasta in a huge bowl. Add the avocado, basil, and tomatoes and mix until thoroughly blended.

2.   Whisk the oil, lime juice, agave syrup, and sea salt in a deep mixing pot. Toss over the pasta, then stir to blend.

Nutrition

Calories: 491 Carbs: 50g Fat: 26g Protein: 15g

The Grilled Romaine Lettuce Salad

Preparation Time: 15 minutes | **Cooking Time**: 10 minutes | **Servings**: 3

Ingredients:

o   4 small heads romaine lettuce, rinsed

o   1 tbsp. red onion, chopped finely

o   1 tbsp. key lime juice

o   Onion powder, to taste

o   1 tbsp. fresh basil, chopped

o   Sea salt and cayenne pepper, to taste

o   4 tbsp. olive oil

o   1 tbsp. agave syrup

Directions:

1.   Place halves of lettuce in a broad non-stick pan cut side down. Do not add oil. Observe the lettuce color by turning them around. Check that the lettuce browns on both faces.

2.   Take off the pan from heat and let the lettuce cool down on a broad platter.

3.   In a small mixing pot, add red onion and olive oil, agave syrup, key lime juice, and fresh basil for dressing. Sprinkle with salt and cayenne pepper. Whisk to blend correctly.

4.   Transfer grilled lettuce and drizzle with the dressing onto a serving plate. Enjoy it!

Nutrition

Calories: 15 Carbs: 3g Fat: 0g Protein: 1g

Alkaline Vegan Salad

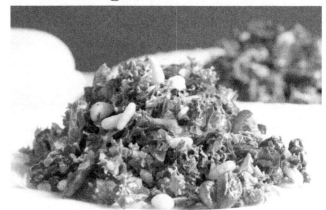

Preparation Time: 5 minutes | **Cooking Time**: 0 minutes | **Servings**: 1

Ingredients:

o   1 small head of lettuce, cut thinly

o   1 medium-sized onion, chopped into small pieces

o   10 plum tomatoes, cut into small pieces

o   Juice of 1 orange

o   1/2 cucumber, spiraled, cut into small pieces, or sliced

o   1/2 apple peeled and diced

o   1/2 teaspoon cayenne pepper

o   A pinch of salt

Directions:

1. Put everything into a bowl and uniformly blend.
2. You may consume it as is or apply a homemade dressing, tahini, or hummus to the salad.

Nutrition

Calories: 290 Carbs: 18g Fat: 19g Protein: 10g

Onion Avocado Salad

Preparation Time: 15 minutes | **Cooking Time**: 0 minutes | **Servings**: 1

Ingredients:

o 1 avocado diced or chopped into small pieces

o 2 medium-sized onion, sliced or diced

o 6 to 8 cherry or plum tomatoes, sliced or diced

o 1 tsp lime juice (optional)

o A pinch of sea salt (optional)

o 1/2 tsp cayenne pepper

Directions:

1. In a pot, add the onion, avocado, and tomato and blend well to mix. Add lime juice, sea salt, then cayenne, then toss.
2. You may eat this salad by itself or with vegetables, cooked quinoa, spelt dumplings, or some other alternative of your preference.

Nutrition:

Calories: 201 Carbs: 12g Fat: 18g Protein: 2g

Mushroom Cucumber Salad

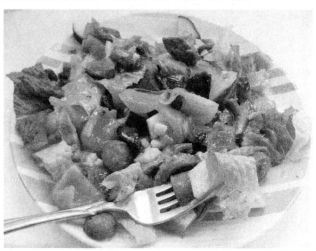

Preparation Time: 15 minutes | **Cooking Time**: 0 minutes | **Servings**: 1

Ingredients:

o 5 Medium-sized Mushrooms (diced)

o 2 Lettuce Leaves (chopped, thinly)

o 1/2 Cucumber (peeled and shred with a peeler to get thin slices)

o Orange Juice (juice of half of a small orange)

o 1 Tbsp Mixed Dried Herbs

o 1/4 Tsp Salt

o 2 Tbsp Lime/Lemon Juice

o 5 Cherry or Plum Tomatoes (chopped)

o 1/2 Tbsp Cayenne Pepper (or Black Pepper)

Directions:

1. Combine all ingredients in a salad bowl and combine to ensure a nice mixture of all.
2. You can get your salad straight away or place it in the fridge for at least an hour to marinate the flavors.

Nutrition

Calories: 100 Carbs: 8g Fat: 1g Protein: 1g

Mushroom Tomato Salad

Preparation Time: 15 minutes | **Cooking Time**: 0 minutes | **Servings**: 1

Ingredients:

o 1 Small Tangerine juice

o 2 Stalks Scallion/spring onions, diced

- o 6 Medium-sized mushrooms, diced
- o 6 Cherry or plum tomatoes, cut in quarters
- o 2 Spring Coriander/ cilantro, diced
- o 1/2 Medium lime or 1 small lime juice
- o 1 Tsp Dried herbs
- o 1 Tsp Olive oil
- o 1/2 Tsp Turmeric
- o 1/2 Tsp Cayenne pepper
- o 1/2 Tsp Sea salt

Directions:
1. In a bowl, mix mushroom, tomato, scallion, cilantro, and toss 2. Add olive oil, lime juice, dried herbs, then mix 3. Add tangerine juice and mix.
2. Let it cool within an hour on the counter or refrigerate for a longer duration. If you choose, you may use salad dressing, but this is not required. Use it as your side meal or main course.

Nutrition
Calories: 222 Carbs: 31g Fat: 0g Protein: 15g

Pasta Salad

Preparation Time: 15 minutes | **Cooking Time**: 15 minutes | **Servings**: 4

Ingredients:
- o 2 boxes of spelt penne
- o 2 avocados cut into small pieces
- o 1/2 cup of chopped onions
- o 1/4 cup of almond milk
- o 1/4 cup of fresh lime juice
- o 3 tbs of maple syrup
- o 1 1/2 cup of sun-dried tomatoes
- o 4 tbs of sea salt
- o 3-4 dashes of cilantro
- o 1/2 cup of olive oil

Directions:
1. Cook the pasta as per the instructions.

2. Add all the fixings in a big bowl. Mix until evenly distributed.
3. Serve.

Nutrition:
Calories: 251 Carbs: 30g Fat: 9g Protein: 11g

Easy Salad

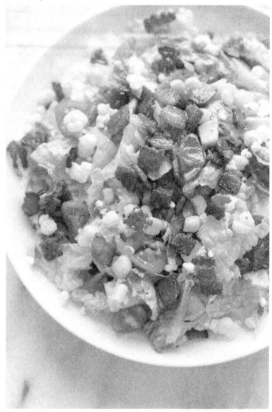

Preparation Time: 5 minutes | **Cooking Time**: 0 minutes | **Servings**: 1

Ingredients:
- o 6 lettuce leaves
- o 6 cherry or plum tomatoes, chopped
- o 3-4 mushrooms, chopped
- o 1/2 cucumber, chopped
- o 10 olives
- o Juice of half of a lime
- o 1 tsp coconut oil/olive oil (optional)

Directions:
1. Put the lettuce in a bowl, break it with your hand into pieces. Add mushroom, sliced tomatoes, and cucumber. Mix all up.

2. Add olives, lime juice, cold-pressed oil, and salt. Mix all up. They are ready to eat.

Nutrition

Calories: 110 Carbs: 4g Fat: 9g Protein: 4g

Salad Alkaline Electric Recipe

Preparation Time: 5 minutes | **Cooking Time**: 0 minutes | **Servings**: 1

Ingredients:

o   Romaine Lettuce

o   1 Kale

o   4 Roma Tomatoes

o   1 Yellow Pepper

o   1 Orange Pepper

o   2 Red Onion

o   3 Jalapeno

o   Extra Virgin Olive Oil (Apply as desired)

o   Apple Cider Vinegar (Optional)

Directions:

1. Rinse and dry all the Ingredients. Chop the Ingredients

2. Place them in a bowl. Sprinkle extra virgin olive oil. Optional: Add Apple Cider Vinegar.

Nutrition:

Calories: 100 Carbs: 0g Fat: 0g Protein: 0g

Simple Fruit Salad

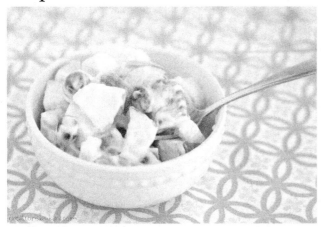

Preparation Time: 5 minutes | **Cooking Time**: 0 minutes | **Servings**: 1

Ingredients:

o   1 banana

o   1 persimmon

o   1 mango

o   1 apple

o   6 – 7 dates

Directions:

1. Wash and slice apple, mango then persimmon, then mix in a bowl.

2. Peel and cut banana, add with date in a bowl.

Nutrition:

Calories: 120 Carbs: 31g Fat: 1g Protein: 1g

Mushroom Salad

Preparation Time: 30 minutes | **Cooking Time**: 0 minutes | **Servings**: 1

Ingredients:

o   1/4 bunch fresh spinach, torn

o   1/4 bunch red leaf lettuce, torn

o   1/4 bunch romaine lettuce, torn

o   1/2 lb. fresh mushrooms

o   1/2 red bell pepper, chopped

o   1 sm. red onion, diced

o   1/2 cup olive oil

o   1/4 cup fresh lime juice

o   1/2 tsp. dill

o   1/2 tsp. basil

o   1/2 tsp. sea salt

Directions:

1. Thoroughly wash mushrooms, dry, slice Add onion, bell pepper, olive oil, lime juice, dill, sea salt, and basil

2. Marinade 1/2 hour in the refrigerator Thoroughly wash greens, dry and shred

3. Place greens with mushrooms and mix them thoroughly. Enjoy!

Nutrition:

Calories: 70 Carbs: 1g Fat: 3g Protein: 1g

Rosemary Carrots Mix

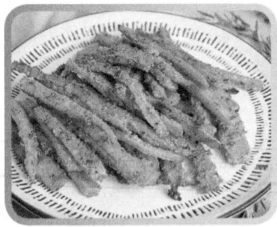

Preparation Time: 10 minutes | **Cooking Time**: 40 minutes | **Servings**: 6

Ingredients:

o   15 carrots, halved lengthwise

o   ¼ cup avocado oil

o   ½ teaspoon rosemary, dried

o   ½ teaspoon garlic powder

o   A pinch of black pepper

Directions:

1.   In a roasting pan, mix the carrots with the oil and the other Ingredients, put in the oven.

2.   Bake at 400 F within 40 minutes.

3.   Serve.

Nutrition

Calories 211 Fat 2g Fiber 6g Carbs 14g Protein 8g

Thai Quinoa Salad

Preparation time: 10 minutes | **Cooking time**: 0 minutes | **Servings**: 1-2

Ingredients:

Ingredients used for dressing:

o   1 tbsp. Sesame seed

o   1 tsp. Chopped garlic

o   1 tsp. Lemon, fresh juice

o   3 tsp. Apple Cider Vinegar

o   2 tsp. Tamari, gluten-free.

o   1/4 cup of tahini (sesame butter)

o   1 pitted date

o   1/2 tsp. Salt

o   1/2 tsp. toasted Sesame oil

Salad Ingredients:

o   1 cup of quinoa, steamed

o   1 big handful of arugulas

o   1 tomato cut in pieces

o   1/4 of the red onion, diced

Directions:

1.   Add the following to a small blender: 1/4 cup + 2 tbsp.

2.   Filtered water, the rest of the ingredients. Blend, man. Steam 1 cup of quinoa in a steamer or a rice pan, then set aside.

3.   Combine the quinoa, the arugula, the tomatoes sliced, the red onion diced on a serving plate or bowl, add the Thai dressing

4.   and serve with a spoon.

Nutrition

Calories: 100 Carbohydrates: 12 g

Green Goddess Bowl and Avocado Cumin Dressing

Preparation time: 10 minutes | **Cooking time**: 0 minutes | **Servings**: 1-2

Ingredients:

Ingredients for the dressing of avocado cumin:

o   1 Avocado

o   1 tbsp. Cumin Powder

o   2 limes, freshly squeezed

o   1 cup of filtered water

o   1/4 seconds. sea salt

o   1 tbsp. Olive extra virgin olive oil

o   Cayenne pepper dash

o   Optional: 1/4 tsp. Smoked pepper

Tahini Lemon Dressing Ingredients:

o   1/4 cup of tahini (sesame butter)

o   1/2 cup of filtered water (more if you want thinner, less thick)

o   1/2 lemon, freshly squeezed

o   1 clove of minced garlic

o   3/4 tsp. Sea salt (Celtic Gray, Himalayan, Redmond Real Salt)

o   1 tbsp. Olive extra virgin olive oil

o   black pepper taste

Salad Ingredients:

o   3 cups of kale, chopped

o   1/2 cup of broccoli flowers, chopped

o   1/2 zucchini (make spiral noodles)

o   1/2 cup of kelp noodles, soaked and drained

o   1/3 cup of cherry tomatoes, halved.

o   2 tsp. hemp seeds

Directions:

1.   Gently steam the kale and the broccoli (flash the steam for 4 minutes), set aside.

2.   Mix the zucchini noodles and kelp noodles and toss with a generous portion of the smoked avocado cumin dressing. Add the cherry tomatoes and stir again.

3.   Place the steamed kale and broccoli and drizzle with the lemon tahini dressing. Top the kale and the broccoli with the noodles and tomatoes and sprinkle the whole dish with the hemp seeds.

Nutrition:

Calories: 89 Carb: 11g Fat: 1.2g Protein: 4g

Sweet And Savory Salad

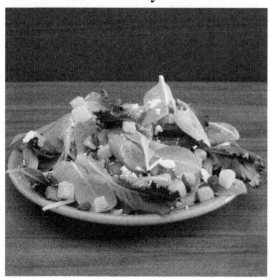

Preparation time: 10 minutes | **Cooking time**: 0 minutes | **Servings**: 1-2

Ingredients:

o   1 big head of butter lettuce

o   1/2 of cucumber, sliced

o   1 pomegranate, seed or 1/3 cup of seed

o   1 avocado, 1 cubed

o   1/4 cup of shelled pistachio, chopped

Ingredients for dressing.

o   1/4 cup of apple cider vinegar

o   1/2 cup of olive oil

o   1 clove of garlic, minced

Directions:

1.   Put the butter lettuce in a salad bowl.

2.   Add the remaining Ingredients and toss with the salad dressing.

Nutrition:

Calories: 68 Carb: 8g Fat: 1.2g Protein: 2g

Kale Pesto's Pasta

Preparation time: 10 minutes | **Cooking time**: 0 minutes | **Servings**: 1-2

Ingredients:

o   1 bunch of kale

o   2 cups of fresh basil

o   1/4 cup of extra virgin olive oil

o   1/2 cup of walnuts

o   2 limes, freshly squeezed

o   Sea salt and chili pepper

o   1 zucchini, noodle (spiralizer)

o   Optional: garnish with chopped asparagus, spinach leaves, and tomato

Directions:

1.   The night before, soak the walnuts to improve absorption.

2.   Put all the recipe ingredients in a blender and blend until the consistency of the cream is reached.

3.   Add the zucchini noodles and enjoy.

Nutrition

Calories: 55 Carbohydrates: 9 g Fat: 1.2g

Beet Salad with Basil Dressing

Preparation time: 10 minutes | **Cooking time**: 0 minutes | **Servings**: 4

Ingredients:

Ingredients for the dressing

o ¼ cup blackberries

o ¼ cup extra-virgin olive oil

o Juice of 1 lemon

o 2 tablespoons minced fresh basil

o 1 teaspoon poppy seeds

o A pinch of sea salt

o For the salad

o 2 celery stalks, chopped

o 4 cooked beets, peeled and chopped

o 1 cup blackberries

o 4 cups spring mix

Directions:

1. To make the dressing, mash the blackberries in a bowl. Whisk in the oil, lemon juice, basil, poppy seeds, and sea salt.
2. To make the salad: Add the celery, beets, blackberries, and spring mix to the bowl with the dressing.
3. Combine and serve.

Nutrition:

Calories: 192   Fats: 15g   Carbs: 15g   Proteins: 2g

Basic Salad with Olive Oil Dressing

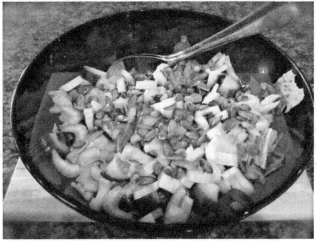

Preparation time: 10 minutes | **Cooking time**: 0 minute | **Servings**: 4

Ingredients:

o 1 cup coarsely chopped iceberg lettuce

o 1 cup coarsely chopped romaine lettuce

o 1 cup fresh baby spinach

o 1 large tomato, hulled and coarsely chopped

o 1 cup diced cucumber

o 2 tablespoons extra-virgin olive oil

o ¼ teaspoon of sea salt

Directions:

1. In a bowl, combine the spinach and lettuces. Add the tomato and cucumber.
2. Drizzle with oil and sprinkle with sea salt.
3. Mix and serve.

Nutrition:

Calories: 77 Fat: 4g Carbohydrates: 3g Protein: 1g

Spinach & Orange Salad with Oil Drizzle

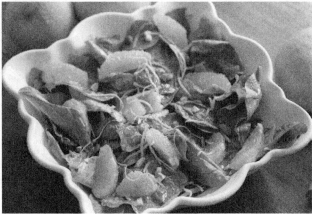

Preparation time: 10 minutes | **Cooking time**: 0 minute **Servings**: 4

Ingredients:

o   4 cups fresh baby spinach

o   1 blood orange, coarsely chopped

o   ½ red onion, thinly sliced

o   ½ shallot, finely chopped

o   2 tbsp. minced fennel fronds

o   Juice of 1 lemon

o   1 tbsp. extra-virgin olive oil

o   Pinch sea salt

Directions:

1.   In a bowl, toss together the spinach, orange, red onion, shallot, and fennel fronds.

2.   Add the lemon juice, oil, and sea salt.

3.   Mix and serve.

Nutrition:

Calories: 79 Fat: 2g Carbohydrates: 8g Protein: 1g

Fruit Salad with Coconut-Lime Dressing

Preparation time: 5 minutes | **Cooking time**: 0 minutes | **Servings**: 4

Ingredients:

Ingredients for the dressing

o   ¼ cup full-fat canned coconut milk

o   1 tbsp. raw honey

o   Juice of ½ lime

o   Pinch sea salt

o   For the salad

o   2 bananas, thinly sliced

o   2 mandarin oranges, segmented

o   ½ cup strawberries, thinly sliced

o   ½ cup raspberries

o   ½ cup blueberries

Directions:

1.   To make the dressing: whisk all the dressing ingredients in a bowl.

2.   To make the salad: Add the salad ingredients in a bowl and mix.

3.   Drizzle with the dressing and serve.

Nutrition:

Calories: 141 Fat: 3g Carb: 30g Protein: 2g

Cranberry And Brussels Sprouts With Dressing

Preparation time: 10 minutes | **Cooking time**: 0 minute | **Servings**: 4

Ingredients:

Ingredients for the dressing

o   ⅓ cup extra-virgin olive oil

o   2 tbsp. apple cider vinegar

o   1 tbsp. pure maple syrup

o   Juice of 1 orange

o   ½ tbsp. dried rosemary

o   1 tbsp. scallion, whites only

o   Pinch sea salt

For the salad

o   1 bunch scallions, greens only, finely chopped

o   1 cup Brussels sprouts, stemmed, halved, and thinly sliced

o   ½ cup fresh cranberries

o   4 cups fresh baby spinach

Directions:

1.   To make the dressing: In a bowl, whisk the dressing ingredients.

2. To make the salad: Add the scallions, Brussels sprouts, cranberries, and spinach to the bowl with the dressing.

3. Combine and serve.

Nutrition:

Calories: 267 Fat: 18g Carb: 26g Protein: 2g

Parsnip, Carrot, And Kale Salad with Dressing

Preparation time: 10 minutes | **Cooking time**: 0 minutes | **Servings**: 4

Ingredients:

Ingredients for the dressing

o ⅓ cup extra-virgin olive oil

o Juice of 1 lime

o 2 tbsp. minced fresh mint leaves

o 1 tsp. pure maple syrup

o Pinch sea salt

For the salad

o 1 bunch kale, chopped

o ½ parsnip, grated

o ½ carrot, grated

o 2 tbsp. sesame seeds

Directions:

1. To make the dressing, mix all the dressing ingredients in a bowl.

2. To make the salad, add the kale to the dressing and massage the dressing into the kale for 1 minute.

3. Add the parsnip, carrot, and sesame seeds.

4. Combine and serve.

Nutrition

Calories: 214 Fat: 2g Carb: 12g Protein: 2g

Tomato Toasts

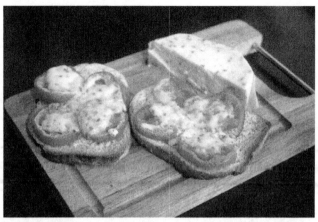

Preparation time: 5 minutes | **Cooking time**: 5 minutes | **Servings**: 4

Ingredients:

o 4 slices of sprouted bread toasts

o 2 tomatoes, sliced

o 1 avocado, mashed

o 1 teaspoon olive oil

o 1 pinch of salt

o ¾ teaspoon ground black pepper

Directions:

1. Blend together the olive oil, mashed avocado, salt, and ground black pepper.

2. When the mixture is homogenous – spread it over the sprouted bread.

3. Then place the sliced tomatoes over the toasts.

4. Enjoy!

Nutrition

Calories: 125 Fat: 11.1g Carbohydrates: 7.0g Protein: 1.5g

Everyday Salad

Preparation time: 10 minutes | **Cooking time**: 40 minutes | **Servings**: 6

Ingredients:

o 5 halved mushrooms

o 6 halved Cherry (Plum) Tomatoes

o 6 rinsed Lettuce Leaves

o 10 olives

o ½ chopped cucumber

o   Juice from ½ Key Lime

o   1 teaspoon olive oil

o   Pure Sea Salt

Directions:

1. Tear rinsed lettuce leaves into medium pieces and put them in a medium salad bowl.
2. Add mushrooms halves, chopped cucumber, olives, and cherry tomato halves into the bowl. Mix well. Pour olive and Key Lime juice over salad.
3. Add pure sea salt to taste. Mix it all till it is well combined.

Nutrition

Calories: 88 Carbs: 11g Fat: .5g Protein: .8g

Sebi's Vegetable Salad

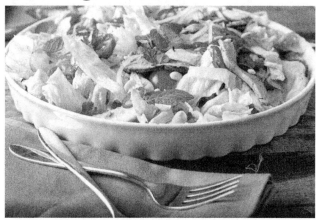

Preparation time: 10 minutes | **Cooking time**: 0 minutes | **Servings**: 1-2

Ingredients:

o   4 cups each of raw spinach and romaine lettuce

o   2 cups each of cherry tomatoes, sliced cucumber, chopped baby carrots, and chopped red, orange, and yellow bell pepper

o   1 cup each of chopped broccoli, sliced yellow squash, zucchini, and cauliflower.

Directions:

1. Wash all these vegetables.
2. Mix in a large mixing bowl and top off with a non-fat or low-fat dressing of your choice.

Nutrition

Calories : 48 Carbohydrates : 11g Protein : 3g

Dessert and Snack Recipes

Chocolate Crunch Bars

Preparation Time: 3 hours | **Cooking Time:** 5 minutes | **Servings:** 4

Ingredients:

o 1 1/2 cups sugar-free chocolate chips

o 1 cup walnut butter

o Stevia to taste

o 1/4 cup coconut oil

o 3 cups pecans, chopped

Directions:

1. Layer an 8-inch baking pan with parchment paper.
2. Mix chocolate chips with butter, coconut oil, and sweetener in a bowl.
3. Melt it by heating in a microwave for 2 to 3 minutes until well mixed.
4. Stir in nuts and seeds. Mix gently.
5. Pour this batter into the baking pan and spread evenly.
6. Refrigerate for 2 to 3 hours.
7. Slice and serve.

Nutrition

Calories: 316 Fat: 30.9g Carbs: 8.3g Protein: 6.4g Fiber: 3.8g

Walnut butter Bars

Preparation Time: 40 minutes | **Cooking Time:** 10 minutes | **Servings:** 6

Ingredients:

o 3/4 cup coconut flour

o 2 oz. walnut butter

o 1/4 cup Swerve

o 1/2 cup walnut butter

o 1/2 teaspoon vanilla

Directions:

1. Combine all the ingredients for bars.
2. Transfer this mixture to 6-inch small pan. Press it firmly.
3. Refrigerate for 30 minutes.
4. Slice and serve.

Nutrition

Calories: 214 Fat: 19g Carbs: 6.5g Protein: 6.5g Fiber: 2.1g

Homemade Protein Bar

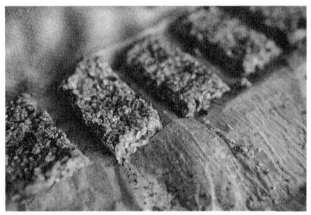

Preparation Time: 5 minutes | **Cooking Time:** 10 minutes | **Servings:** 4

Ingredients:

o 1 cup walnut butter

o 4 tablespoons coconut oil

o 2 scoops vanilla protein

o Stevia, to taste

o ½ teaspoon sea salt

o Optional Ingredients:

o 1 teaspoon cinnamon

Directions:

1. Mix coconut oil with butter, protein, stevia, and salt in a dish.
2. Stir in cinnamon and chocolate chip.
3. Press the mixture firmly and freeze until firm.
4. Cut the crust into small bars.

5. Serve and enjoy.

Nutrition
Calories: 179 Fat: 15.7g Carbs: 4.8g Protein: 5.6g
Fiber: 0.8g

Shortbread Cookies

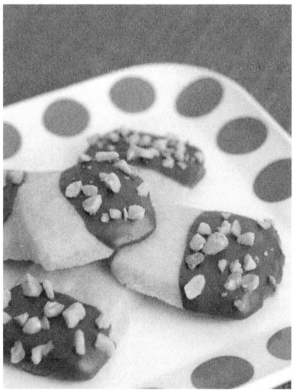

Preparation Time: 10 minutes | **Cooking Time:**
1 hour 10 minutes | **Servings:** 6
Ingredients:

o   2 1/2 cups coconut flour

o   6 tablespoons walnut butter

o   1/2 cup erythritol

o   1 teaspoon vanilla essence

Directions:

1. Preheat your oven to 350 degrees F.
2. Layer a cookie sheet with parchment paper.
3. Beat butter with erythritol until fluffy.
4. Stir in vanilla essence and coconut flour. Mix well until crumbly.
5. Spoon out a tablespoon of cookie dough onto the cookie sheet.
6. Add more dough to make as many cookies as possible.

7. Bake for 15 minutes until brown.
8. Serve.

Nutrition
Calories: 288 Fat: 25.3g Carbs: 9.6g Protein: 7.6g
Fiber: 3.8g

Coconut Chip Cookies

Preparation Time: 10 minutes**Cooking Time:** 15
minutes**Servings:** 4
Ingredients:

o   1 cup coconut flour

o   ½ cup cacao nibs

o   ½ cup coconut flakes, unsweetened

o   1/3 cup erythritol

o   ½ cup walnut butter

o   ¼ cup walnut butter, melted

o   ¼ cup coconut milk

o   Stevia, to taste

o   ¼ teaspoon sea salt

Directions:

1. Preheat your oven to 350 degrees F.
2. Layer a cookie sheet with parchment paper.
3. Add and combine all the dry ingredients in a glass bowl.
4. Whisk in butter, coconut milk, vanilla essence, stevia, and walnut butter.
5. Beat well then stir in dry mixture. Mix well.
6. Spoon out a tablespoon of cookie dough on the cookie sheet.
7. Add more dough to make as many as 16 cookies.
8. Flatten each cookie using your fingers.
9. Bake for 25 minutes until golden brown.
10. Let them sit for 15 minutes.
11. Serve.

Nutrition:
Calories: 192 Fat: 17.44g Carbs: 2.2g Protein: 4.7g
Fiber: 2.1g

Coconut Cookies

Preparation Time: 10 minutes | **Cooking Time:** 20 minutes | **Servings:** 6

Ingredients:

o   6 tablespoons coconut flour

o   ¾ teaspoons baking powder

o   1/8 teaspoon sea salt

o   3 tablespoons walnut butter

o   1/6 cup coconut oil

o   6 tablespoon date sugar

o   1/3 cup coconut milk

o   1/2 teaspoon vanilla essence

Directions:

1.   Preheat your oven to 375 degrees F. Layer a cookie sheet with parchment paper.

2.   Beat all the wet ingredients in a mixer. Mix all the dry mixture in a blender.

3.   Stir in the wet mixture and mix well until smooth.

4.   Spoon a tablespoon of cookie dough on the cookie sheet.

5.   Add more dough to make as many cookies as possible. Bake until golden brown (about 10 minutes).

6.   Serve.

Nutrition

Calories: 151 Fat: 13.4g Carbs: 6.4g Protein: 4.2g Fiber: 4.8g

Berry Mousse

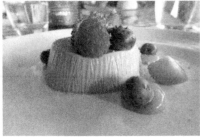

Preparation Time: 5 minutes | **Cooking Time:** 5 minutes | **Servings:** 2

Ingredients:

o   1 teaspoon Seville orange zest

o   3 oz. raspberries or blueberries

o   ¼ teaspoon vanilla essence

o   2 cups coconut cream

Directions:

1.   Blend cream in an electric mixer until fluffy.

2.   Stir in vanilla and Seville orange zest. Mix well.

3.   Fold in nuts and berries.

4.   Cover the bowl with a plastic wrap.

5.   Refrigerate for 3 hours.

6.   Garnish as desired.

7.   Serve.

Nutrition

Calories: 265 Fat: 13g Carbs: 7.5g Protein: 5.2g Fiber: 0.5g

Coconut Pulp Cookies

Preparation Time: 5 minutes | **Cooking Time:** 10 hours | **Servings:** 4

Ingredients:

o   3 cups coconut pulp

o   1 Granny Smith apple

o   1-2 teaspoon cinnamon

o   2-3 tablespoons raw honey

o   1/4 cup coconut flakes

Directions:

1.   Blend coconut pulp with remaining ingredients in a food processor.

2.   Make small cookies out this mixture.

3.   Place them on a cookie sheet, lined with parchment paper.

4.   Place the sheet in a food dehydrator for 6 to 10 hours at 115 degrees F.

5.   Serve.

Nutrition

Calories: 240 Fat: 22.5g Carbs: 17.3g Protein: 14.9g Fiber: 0g

Avocado Pudding

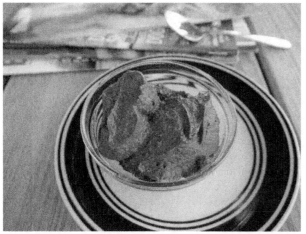

Preparation Time: 10 minutes | **Cooking Time:** 0 minutes | **Servings:** 2

Ingredients:

o   2 avocados

o   3/4-1 cup coconut milk

o   1/3-1/2 cup raw cacao powder

o   1 trasponi 100% pure organici vacilla (optional)

o   2-4 tablespoons date sugar

Directions:

1.   Blend all the ingredients in a blender.
2.   Refrigerate for 4 hours in a container.
3.   Serve.

Nutrition

Calories: 609 Fat: 50.5g Carbs: 9.9g Protein: 29.3g Fiber: 1.5g

Coconut Raisins cookies

Preparation Time: 10 minutes | **Cooking Time:** 10 minutes | **Servings:** 4

Ingredients:

o   1 1/4 cup coconut flour

o   1 cup walnut flour

o   1 teaspoon baking soda

o   1/2 teaspoon Celtic Sea salt

o   1 cup walnut butter

o   1 cup coconut date sugar

o   2 teaspoons vanilla

o   ¼ cup coconut milk

o   3/4 cup organic raisins

o   3/4 cup coconut chips or flakes

Directions:

1.   Set your oven to 357 degrees F.
2.   Mix flour with salt and baking soda.
3.   Blend butter with sugar until creamy then stirs in coconut milk and vanilla.
4.   Mix well then stir in dry mixture. Mix until smooth.
5.   Fold in all the remaining ingredients.
6.   Make small cookies out this dough.
7.   Arrange the cookies on a baking sheet.
8.   Bake for 10 minutes until golden brown.

Nutrition

Calories: 237 Fat: 19.8g Carbs: 55.1g Protein: 17.8g Fiber: 0.9g

Zucchini Chips

Preparation Time: 5 minutes | **Cooking Time:** 12 minutes | **Servings:** 4

Ingredients:

o   4 zucchinis, washed, peeled, and sliced

o   2 teaspoons extra-virgin olive oil

o   1/4 teaspoon sea salt

Directions:

1.   Set your oven to 350 degrees F.
2.   Toss zucchinis with salt and olive oil.
3.   Spread the slices on two baking sheets in a single layer.
4.   Bake for 6 minutes on upper and lower rack of the oven.
5.   Switch the baking racks and bake for another 6 minutes.
6.   Serve.

Nutrition

Calories: 153 Fat: 7.5g Carbs: 20.4g Protein: 3.1g Fiber: 0g

Spinach and Sesame

Preparation Time: 5 minutes | **Cooking Time:** 15 minutes | **Servings:** 4

Ingredients:

o   2 tablespoons white sesame seeds

o   1 cup fresh spinach, washed

o   1 2/3 cups all-purpose flour

o   1/2 cup water

o   1/2 teaspoon baking powder

o   1 teaspoon olive oil

o   1 teaspoon salt

Directions:

1. Transfer the spinach to a blender with a half cup of water and blend until smooth.

2. Add 2 tablespoons white sesame seeds, 1/2 teaspoon baking powder, 1 2/3 cups all-purpose flour, and 1 teaspoon salt to a bowl and stir well until combined. Add in 1 teaspoon olive oil and spinach water. Mix again and knead by using your hands until you obtain a smooth dough.

3. If the made dough is too gluey, then add more flour.

4. Using your parchment paper, lightly roll out the dough as thin as possible. Cut into squares with a pizza cutter.

5. Bake in a preheated oven at 400°, for about 15to 20 minutes. Once done, let cool and then serve.

Nutrition

Calories: 223 Fat: 3g Total Carbohydrates: 41g Protein: 6g

Mini Nacho Pizzas

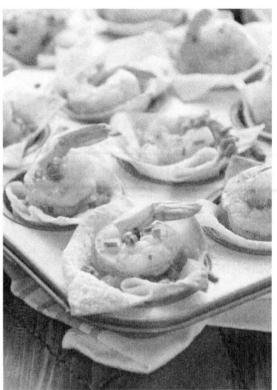

Preparation Time: 5 minutes | **Cooking Time:** 10 minutes | **Servings:** 4

Ingredients:

o   1/4 cup refried beans, vegan

o   2 tablespoons tomato, diced

o   2 English muffins split in half

o   1/4 cup onion, sliced

o   1/3 cup vegan cheese, shredded

o   1 small jalapeno, sliced

o   1/3 cup roasted tomato salsa

o   1/2 avocado, diced and tossed in lemon juice

Directions:

1. Add the refried beans/salsa onto the muffin bread. Sprinkle with shredded vegan cheese, followed by the veggie toppings.

2. Transfer to baking sheet & place in a preheated oven at 350 to 400 F on a top rack.

3. Put into the oven for 10 minutes and then broil for 2 minutes so that the top becomes bubbly.

4. Take out from oven & let them cool at room temperature.

5. Top with avocado. Enjoy!

Nutrition

Calories: 133 Fat: 4.2g Carbs: 719g Protein: 6g

Pizza Sticks

Preparation Time: 10 minutes | **Cooking Time:** 30 minutes | **Servings:** 16 sticks

Ingredients:

o   5 tablespoons tomato sauce

o   Few pinches of dried basil

o   1 block extra firm tofu

o   2 tablespoons

o   2 teaspoons Nutritional yeast

Directions:

1.   Cape the tofu in a paper tissue, put a cutting board on top, and place something heavy on top and drain for about 10 to 15 minutes.

2.   In the meantime, line your baking sheet with parchment paper. Cut the tofu into 16 equal pieces and place them on a baking sheet.

3.   Spread each pizza stick with a teaspoon of marinara sauce.

4.   Sprinkle each stick with a half teaspoon of yeast, followed by basil on top.

5.   Bake in a preheated oven at 425 F for about 28 to 30 minutes. Serve and enjoy!

Nutrition

Calories: 33 Fat: 1.7g Total Carbs: 2g Protein: 3g

Raw Broccoli Poppers

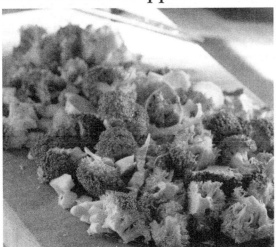

Preparation Time: 2 minutes | **Cooking Time:** 8 minutes | **Servings:** 4

Ingredients:

o   1/8 cup water

o   1/8 teaspoon fine sea salt

o   4 cups broccoli florets, washed and cut into 1-inch pieces

o   1/4 teaspoon turmeric powder

o   1 cup unsalted cashews, soaked overnight or at least 3-4 hours and drained

o   1/4 teaspoon onion powder

o   1 red bell pepper, seeded and

o   2 heaping tablespoons Nutritional

o   2 tablespoons lemon juice

Directions:

1.   Transfer the drained cashews to a high-speed blender and pulse for about 30 seconds. Add in the chopped pepper and pulse again for 30seconds.

2.   Add some 2 tablespoons lemon juice, 1/8 cup water, 2heaping tablespoons Nutritional yeast, 1/4 teaspoon onion powder, 1/8 teaspoon fine sea salt, and 1/4 teaspoon turmeric powder. Pulse for about 45 seconds until smooth.

3.   Handover the broccoli into a bowl and add in chopped cheesy cashew mixture. Toss well until coated.

4.   Transfer the pieces of broccoli to the trays of a yeast dehydrator.

5.   Follow the dehydrator's instructions and dehydrate for about 8 minutes at 125 F or until crunchy.

Nutrition

Calories: 408 Fat: 32g Total Carbohydrates: 22g Protein: 15g

Blueberry Cauliflower

Preparation Time: 2 minutes | **Cooking Time:** 5 minutes | **Servings:** 1

Ingredients:

o   1/4 cup frozen strawberries

o   2 teaspoons maple syrup

o   3/4 cup unsweetened cashew milk

- o 1 teaspoon vanilla extract
- o 1/2 cup plain cashew yogurt
- o 5 tablespoons powdered peanut butter
- o 3/4 cup frozen wild blueberries
- o 1/2 cup cauliflower florets, coarsely chopped

Directions:

1. Add all the smoothie ingredients to a high-speed blender.
2. Blitz to combine until smooth.
3. Pour into a chilled glass and serve.

Nutrition

Calories: 340 Fat: 11g Total Carbohydrates: 48g Protein: 16g

Candied Ginger

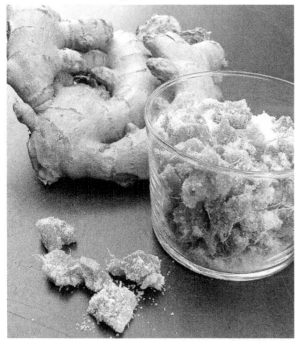

Preparation Time: 10 minutes | **Cooking Time:** 40 minutes | **Servings:** 3 to 5

Ingredients:

- o 2 1/2 cups salted pistachios, shelled
- o 1 1/4 teaspoons powdered ginger
- o 3 tablespoons pure maple syrup

Directions:

1. Add 1 1/4 teaspoons powdered ginger to a bowl with pistachios. Stir well until combined. There
2. Should be no lumps.
3. Drizzle w/ 3 tablespoons of maple syrup and stir well.
4. Transfer to a baking sheet lined with parchment paper and spread evenly.
5. Cook into a preheated oven at 275 F for about 20 minutes.
6. Take out from the oven, stir, and cook for a further 10 to 15 minutes.
7. Let it cool for about a few minutes until crispy. Enjoy!

Nutrition

Calories: 378 Fat: 27.6g Total Carbohydrates: 26g Protein: 13g

Chia Crackers

Preparation Time: 20 minutes | **Cooking Time:** 1 hour

Servings: 24-26 crackers

Ingredients:

- o 1/2 cup pecans, chopped
- o 1/2 cup chia seeds
- o 1/2 teaspoon cayenne pepper
- o 1 cup of water
- o 1/4 cup Nutritional yeast
- o 1/2 cup pumpkin seeds
- o 1/4 cup ground flax
- o Salt and pepper, to taste

Directions:

1. Mix around 1/2 cup chia seeds and 1 cup water. Keep it aside.
2. Take another bowl and combine all the remaining ingredients. Combine well and stir in the chia water mixture until you obtained dough.
3. Transfer dough onto a baking sheet and rollout (1/4" thick).
4. Transfer into a preheated oven at 325°F and bake for about half an hour.

5. Take out from the oven, flip over the dough, and cut it into the desired cracker shape/squares.

6. Spread and back again for a further half an hour, or until crispy and browned.

7. Once done, take them out from the oven and let them cool at room temperature. Enjoy!

Nutrition

Calories: 41 Fat: 3.1g Total Carbohydrates: 2g Protein: 2g

Orange- Spiced Pumpkin Hummus

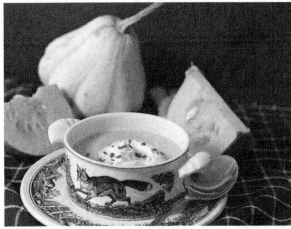

Preparation Time: 2 minutes | **Cooking Time:** 5 minutes | **Servings:** 4 cups

Ingredients:

o 1 tablespoon maple syrup

o 1/2 teaspoon salt

o 1 can (16oz.) garbanzo beans,

o 1/8 teaspoon ginger or nutmeg

o 1 cup canned pumpkin Blend,

o 1/8 teaspoon cinnamon

o 1/4 cup tahini

o 1 tablespoon fresh orange juice

o Pinch of orange zest, for garnish

o 1 tablespoon apple cider vinegar

Directions:

1. Mix all the ingredients to a food processor blender and blend until slightly chunky.

2. Serve right away and enjoy!

Nutrition

Calories: 291 Fat: 22.9g Total Carbohydrates: 15g Protein: 12g

Cinnamon Maple Sweet Potato Bites

Preparation Time: 5 minutes | **Cooking Time:** 25 minutes | **Servings:** 3 to 4

Ingredients:

o 1/2 teaspoon corn-starch

o 1 teaspoon cinnamon

o 4 medium sweet potatoes, then peeled and cut into bite-size cubes

o 2 to 3 tablespoons maple syrup

o 3 tablespoons butter, melted

Directions:

1. Transfer the potato cubes to a Ziploc bag and add in 3 tablespoons of melted butter. Seal and shake well until the potato cubes are coated with butter.

2. Add in the remaining ingredients and shake again.

3. Transfer the potato cubes to a parchment-lined baking sheet. Cubes shouldn't be stacked on one another.

4. If needed, sprinkle with cinnamon and bake in a preheated oven at 425°F for about 25 to 30 minutes, stirring once during cooking.

5. Once done, take them out and stand them at room temperature. Enjoy!

Nutrition

Calories: 436 Fat: 17.4g Total Carbohydrates: 71.8g Protein: 4.1g

Cheesy Kale Chips

Preparation Time: 3 minutes | **Cooking Time:** 12 minutes | **Servings:** 4

Ingredients:

- o   3 tablespoons Nutritional yeast
- o   1 head curly kale, washed, ribs
- o   3/4 teaspoon garlic powder
- o   1 tablespoon olive oil
- o   1 teaspoon onion powder
- o   Salt, to taste.

Directions:

1. Line cookie sheets with parchment paper.
2. Drain the kale leaves and spread on a paper removed and leaves torn into the chip-
3. Towel. Then, kindly transfer the leaves to a bowl and sized pieces
4. add in 1 teaspoon onion powder, 3 tablespoons Nutritional yeast, 1 tablespoon olive oil, and 3/4
5. Teaspoon garlic powder. Mix with your hands.
6. Spread the kale onto prepared cookie sheets. They shouldn't touch each other.
7. Bake in a preheated oven for about 350 F for about 10to 12 minutes.
8. Once crisp, take out from the oven, and sprinkle with a bit of salt. Serve and enjoy!

Nutrition

Calories: 71 Fat: 4g Total Carbohydrates: 5g Protein: 4g

Lemon Roasted Bell Pepper

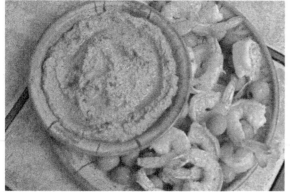

Preparation Time: 10 minutes | **Cooking Time:** 5 minutes | **Servings:** 4

Ingredients:

- o   4 bell peppers
- o   1 teaspoon olive oil

- o   1 tablespoon mango juice
- o   1/4 teaspoon garlic, minced
- o   1 teaspoons oregano
- o   1 pinch salt
- o   1 pinch pepper

Directions:

1. Start heating the Air Fryer to 390 degrees F
2. Place some bell pepper in the Air fryer
3. Drizzle it with the olive oil and air fry for 5 minutes
4. Take a serving plate and transfer it
5. Take a small bowl and add garlic, oregano, mango juice, salt, and pepper
6. Mix them well and drizzle the mixture over the peppers
7. Serve and enjoy!

Nutrition

Calories: 59 Carb: 6 g Fat: 5 g Protein: 4 g

Subtle Roasted Mushrooms

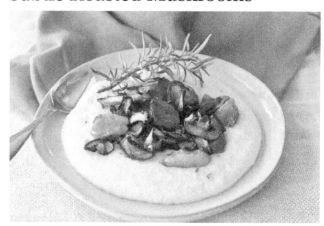

Preparation Time: 10 minutes | **Cooking Time:** 5 minutes | **Servings:** 4

Ingredients:

- o   2 teaspoons mixed Sebi Friendly herbs
- o   1 tablespoon olive oil
- o   1/2 teaspoon garlic powder
- o   2 pounds mushrooms
- o   2 tablespoons date sugar

Directions:

1. Wash mushrooms and turn dry in a plate of mixed greens spinner
2. Quarter them and put them in a safe spot
3. Put garlic, oil, and spices in the dish of your oar type air fryer
4. Warmth for 2 minutes
5. Stir it.
6. Add some mushrooms and cook 25 minutes
7. Then include vermouth and cook for 5 minutes more
8. Serve and enjoy!

Nutrition

Calories: 94 Carb: 3 g Fat: 8 g Protein: 2 g.

Fancy Spelt Bread

Preparation Time: 10 minutes | **Cooking Time:** 5 minutes | **Servings:** 4

Ingredients:

o 1 cup spring water
o 1/2 cup of coconut milk
o 3 tablespoons avocado oil
o 1 teaspoon baking soda
o 1 tablespoon agave nectar
o 4 and 1/2 cups spelt flour
o 1 and 1/2 teaspoon salt

Directions:

1. Preheat your Air Fryer to 355 degrees F
2. Take a big bowl and add baking soda, salt, flour whisk well
3. Add 3/4 cup of water, plus coconut milk, oil and mix well
4. Sprinkle your working surface with flour, add dough to the flour
5. Roll well
6. Knead for about three minutes, adding small amounts of flour until dough is a nice ball
7. Place parchment paper in your cooking basket
8. Lightly grease your pan and put the dough inside
9. Transfer into Air Fryer and bake for 30-45 minutes until done

10. Remove then insert a stick to check for doneness
11. If done already, serve and enjoy; if not, let it cook for a few minutes more

Nutrition

Calories: 203 Carb: 37 g Fat: 4g Protein: 7 g

Crispy Crunchy Hummus

Preparation Time: 10 minutes | **Cooking Time:** 10-15 minutes | **Servings:** 4

Ingredients:

o 1/2 a red onion
o 2 tablespoons fresh coriander
o 1/4 cup cherry tomatoes
o 1/2 a red bell pepper
o 1 tablespoon dulse flakes
o Juice of lime
o Salt to taste
o 3 tablespoons olive oil
o 2 tablespoons tahini
o 1 cup warm chickpeas

Directions:

1. Prepare your Air Fryer cooking basket
2. Add chickpeas to your cooking container and cook for 10-15 minutes, making a point to continue blending them occasionally, until they are altogether warmed
3. Add warmed chickpeas to a bowl and include tahini, salt, lime
4. Utilize a fork to pound chickpeas and fixings in glue until smooth
5. Include hacked onion, cherry tomatoes, ringer pepper, dulse drops, and olive oil
6. Blend well until consolidated
7. Serve hummus with a couple of cuts of spelt bread

Nutrition

Calories: 95 Carb: 5 g Fat: 5 g Protein: 5 g

Pumpkin spice crackers

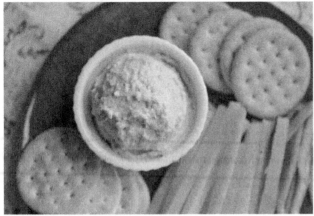

Preparation Time: 10 minutes | **Cooking Time:** 60 minutes | **Servings:** 6

Ingredients:

o   1/3 cup coconut flour

o   2 tablespoons pumpkin pie spice

o   3/4 cup sunflower seeds

o   3/4 cup flaxseed

o   1/3 cup sesame seeds

o   1 tablespoon ground psyllium husk powder

o   1 teaspoon of sea salt

o   3 tablespoons coconut oil, melted

o   11/3 cups alkaline water

Directions:

1.   Set your oven to 300 degrees F.
2.   Combine all dry ingredients in a bowl.
3.   Add water and oil to the mixture and mix well.
4.   Let the dough stay for 2 to 3 mins.
5.   Spread the dough on a cookie sheet lined with parchment paper.
6.   Bake for 30 minutes.
7.   Reduce the oven heat to low and bake for another 30 minutes.
8.   Crack the bread into bite-size pieces.
9.   Serve

Nutrition

Calories: 248 Total Fat: 15.7g Saturated Fat: 2.7g
Cholesterol: 75mg Sodium: 94mg Total Carbs: 0.4g
Fiber: 0g Sugar: 0 g Protein: 24.9 g

Spicy roasted nuts

Preparation Time: 10 minutes | **Cooking Time:** 15 minutes | **Servings:** 4

Ingredients:

o   8 oz. pecans or almonds or walnuts

o   1 teaspoon of sea salt

o   1 tablespoon olive oil or coconut oil

o   1 teaspoon ground cumin

o   1 teaspoon paprika powder or chili powder

Directions:

1.   Add all the ingredients to a skillet.
2.   Roast the nuts until golden brown.
3.   Serve and enjoy.

Nutrition

Calories: 287 Total Fat: 29.5 g Saturated Fat: 3 g
Cholesterol: 0 mg   Total Carbs: 5.9 g   Sugar: 1.4g
Fiber: 4.3 g   Sodium: 388 mg Protein: 4.2 g

Wheat Crackers

Preparation Time: 10 minutes | **Cooking Time:** 20 minutes | **Servings:** 4

Ingredients:

o   1 3/4 cups almond flour

o   1 1/2 cups coconut flour

o   3/4 teaspoon sea salt

o   1/3 cup vegetable oil

o   1 cup alkaline water

o   Sea salt for sprinkling

Directions:

1.   Set your oven to 350 degrees F.
2.   Mix coconut flour, almond flour, and salt in a bowl.
3.   Stir in vegetable oil and water. Mix well until smooth.
4.   Spread this dough on a floured surface into a thin sheet.
5.   Cut small squares out of this sheet.
6.   Arrange the dough squares on a baking sheet lined with parchment paper.
7.   Bake for 20 mins. Until light golden in color.

8. Serve.

Nutrition

Calories: 64 Total Fat: 9.2g Saturated Fat: 2.4g
Cholesterol: 110mg Sodium: 276mg Total Carbs: 9.2g
Fiber: 0.9 g Sugar: 1.4 g   Protein: 1.5 g

Potato Chips

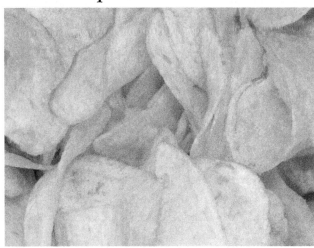

Preparation Time: 10 minutes | **Cooking Time:** 20 minutes | **Servings:** 4

Ingredients:

o   1 tablespoon vegetable oil

o   1 potato, sliced paper thin

o   Sea salt, to taste

Directions:

1. Toss potato with oil and sea salt.
2. Spread the slices in a baking dish in a single layer.
3. Cook in a microwave for 5 minutes until golden brown.
4. Serve.

Nutrition

Calories: 80 Total Fat:3.5g Saturated Fat:0.1 g
Cholesterol: 320mg Sodium: 350mg Total Carbs:11.6g   Fiber: 0.7 g Sugar: 0.7 g Protein: 1.2g

Zucchini Pepper Chips

Preparation Time: 10 minutes | **Cooking Time:** 15 minutes | **Servings:** 4

Ingredients:

o   1 2/3 cups vegetable oil

o   1 teaspoon garlic powder

o   1 teaspoon onion powder

o   1/2 teaspoon black pepper

o   3 tablespoons crushed red pepper flakes

o   2 zucchinis, thinly sliced

Directions:

1. Mix oil with all the spices in a bowl.
2. Add zucchini slices and mix well.
3. Transfer the mixture to a Ziplock bag and seal it.
4. Refrigerate for 10 minutes.
5. Spread the zucchini slices on a greased baking sheet.
6. Bake for 15 minutes
7. Serve.

Nutrition

Calories: 172 Total Fat: 11.1g Saturated Fat: 5.8 g
Cholesterol: 610 mg Sodium: 749 mg
Total Carbs:19.9 g Fiber: 0.2 g Sugar: 0.2 g Protein: 13.5 g

30- Day Meal Plan

Day	Breakfast	Lunch	Dinner	Desserts/Snacks
1	Quinoa Porridge	Chickpea Butternut Squash	Fried Cabbage	Potato Chips
2	Jackfruit Vegetable Fry	Tomato Soup	Pumpkin and White Bean	Chocolate Crunch Bars
3	Flourless Banana Bread	Chickpeas & Squash Stew	Healthy Broccoli Asparagus Soup	Pizza Sticks
4	Amaranth Porridge	Atichoke Sauce Ala Quinoa	Citrus Quinoa with Avocado	Orange-Spiced Pumpkin
5	Scrambled Tofu and Tomato	Spiced Okra	Sweet Potato and Quinoa	Cheesy Kale Chips
6	Squash Hash	Veggie Balls in Tomato Sauce	Mixed Berry-Chia Seed	Candied Ginger
7	Millet Porridge	Zucchini Turnip Soup	Cajun Seasoned Zucchini	Coconut Cookies
8	Hemp Seed Porridge	Yellow Squash & Bell Pepper	Jucama & Sweet Pepper	Pumpkin spice Crackers
9	Thick Alkaline Minestrone	Mushroom Soup	Vanilla Bean and Cinnamon	Francy Spelt Bread
10	Ginger- Sesame Quinoa	Spelt Spaghetti	Whole Cauliflower	Wheat Crackers
11	Crunchy Quinoa Meal	Lentil Kale Soup	Quinoa with Spring	Lemon Roasted Bell Pepper
12	Zucchini Home Fries	The Mysterious Alkaline	Easy Cilantro Lime Quinoa	Spinach and Sesame
13	Ginger-Maple Yam Casserole	Kale, Mushroom, Walnut and Avocado	Oatmeal Porridge	Subtle Roasted Mushrooms
14	Veggie Medley	Quinoa Vegetable Soup	Carrot and Hemp Seed	Coconut Pulp Cookies
15	Zucchini Muffins	Quinoa & Veggie Stew	Sesame and Hemp Seed	Cinnamon Maple Sweet
16	Pumpkin Spice Quinoa	Butternut Squash Plum	Alkaline Pumpkin Coconut	Crispy Crunchy Hummus
17		Mixed Greens Soup	Three Bean Chili	Blueberry Cauliflower
18	Coconut Pancakes	Chickpeas & Kale Stew	Beans and Broccoli in Sauce	Spicy roasted Nuts

19	Butternut Squash, Apple	Veggie Kabobs	Vegetable Stew	Walnut Butter Bars
20	Zucchini Pancakes	Mushroom Curry	Spinach Quinoa	Mini Nacho Pizzas
21	Quinoa Porridge	Mango & Apple Sauce	Cold Cauliflower Coconut	Cinnamon Maple Sweet
22	Scrambled Tofu	Butternut Squash Ginger	Brussels Sprouts & Carrots	Avocado Pudding
23	Sprouted Buckwheat Crepes	Beautifully Curried Eggplant	Tofu Curry	Homemade Protein bar
24	Banana Barley Porridge	Culturally Diverse Pumpkin	Spicy Vegetable Chili	Subtle Roasted Mushrooms
25	Black Berry Pie	Bell Peppers & Zucchini Stir Fry	Alkaline Carrot Soup	Shortbread Cookies
26	Banana Muffins	Turnip Kale Soup	Creamy Asparagus Soup	Raw Broccoli Poppers
27	Vegetarian Pie	Squash&Apple Soup	Sesame Mixed Noodles	Berry Mousse
28	Red Thai Vegetable Curry	Cream of Avocado Mushroom	Alkaline Carrot Soup	Cinnamon Maple Sweet
29	Super Seed Spelt Pancakes	Tomato Sauce	Asparagus Risotto	Zucchini Pepper Chips
30	Breakfast Salad	Coconut Milk and Glazing Stir	Spicy Eggplant	Chia Crackers

Conclusion

Thank you for sticking with me all the way to the end. Diseases are caused by a person being infected by bacteria, viruses, or germs, according to Western medical studies. Inorganic substances are used by physicians to help people resolve this "infestation." Via basic deductive reasoning, Dr. Sebi's study discovered the shortcomings in this premise. These techniques have always been used in Western medicine, and they have always produced the same inadequate results.

Instead, the African approach to illness is diametrically opposed to Western medicine. It denies the existence of bacteria, viruses, and germs. Diseases can expand when the mucous membrane is weakened, according to Dr. Sebi's study. The African Bio-mineral Balance is alkaline since all the compounds are derived from natural plants.

Since viruses can only survive in acidic conditions, this is critical in reversing these pathologies. Since inorganic compounds are acidic, using them to treat diseases makes little sense. The use of natural medicines on a regular basis will detoxify and cleanse a sick body, returning it to an alkaline state.

Dr. Sebi's diet program goes a step further. In addition to removing years of toxin build-up, the African Bio-mineral Balance would replenish all depleted minerals and rejuvenate any acid-damaged cell tissue. The liver, kidneys, gall bladder, colon, and skin are the main organs that it benefits. As toxins are released from one of the organs, they travel around the body and cause disease. Since it is unable to eliminate the poison, the body will eventually target the weakest organ. The colon is one of the essential organs in the body, and it must be cleansed before infections can be reversed.

Every cell in the body will be cleansed by Dr. Sebi's detoxifying cleanse. The body will then regenerate and rejuvenate itself.

The Dr. Sebi diet is an alkaline plant-based diet. It aids in the rejuvenation of the body's cells by removing radioactive waste. A small number of foods, as well as supplements, make up most of the diet.

Dr. Sebi's diet can also help with diseases such as lupus, AIDS, kidney failure, and other illnesses. To cure these diseases, you must consume only certain foods, fruits, and vegetables while strictly avoiding animal products.

This is a very low-protein diet, which is why Dr. Sebi's supplements are so crucial. Soy, animal products, lentils, and beans are not allowed. When it comes to Dr. Sebi's vitamin options, you have many options, including an "all-inclusive" kit that includes 20 different items that will help you restore your body's health.

If you don't want to go for the "all-inclusive" kit, you can choose supplements based on your health concerns. Bio Ferro, for example, can improve overall health, aid digestion, boost immunity, cleanse the blood, treat liver problems, and encourage weight loss.

If you have found this book helpful, I invite you to leave a review directly on the Amazon page. Just scan the QR code on this page with your smartphone.
If you have any other requests or particular questions, you can freely contact me via mail.

scarrett.diet@outlook.com

Remember to also look at my site, I upgrade regulary.

www.suzannescarrett.com

You can also find me on Facebook and if you wish, put a like on my personal page.

Enjoy your life. I wish you much joy and serenity.

Printed in Great Britain
by Amazon

26680303R00066